# ALWAYS

CW01521884

# About The Author

Carolyn Faulder is a medical journalist who began her career on Nova and has contributed features on health and other topics to all the major national newspapers and women's magazines. She is particularly interested in medical ethics and the patient–doctor relationship. Readers may be interested in other titles by the same author:

*Whose Body Is It? The troubling issue of informed consent*
(Virago 1985)

*The Women's Cancer Book*
(Virago 1989)

*A Special Gift: The story of Dr Vicky Clement-Jones
and the foundation of BACUP*
(Michael Joseph 1991)

# ALWAYS A WOMAN

## A Practical Guide To Living With Breast Surgery

*Carolyn Faulder*

Thorsons
*An Imprint of* HarperCollins*Publishers*

Thorsons
An Imprint of HarperCollins*Publishers*
77-85 Fulham Palace Road,
Hammersmith, London W6 8JB

Published by Thorsons 1992
1 3 5 7 9 10 8 6 4 2

© Carolyn Faulder 1992

Carolyn Faulder asserts the moral right to
be identified as the author of this work

A catalogue record for this book
is available from the British Library

ISBN 0 7225 2643 1

Typeset by Harper Phototypesetters Limited
Northampton, England
Printed in Great Britain by
Hartnolls, Bodmin, Cornwall

# Contents

For
Jinty Blanckenhagen
Dr Maureen Roberts
and
Betty Westgate
They cared

# Acknowledgements

My gratitude goes first and foremost to the many women, only some of whom are mentioned by name in this book, who have talked with me about their experience of breast cancer. Each is an individual, so their very different perceptions and their personal reactions have enabled me, I hope, to convey something of what it means to have this disease.

Their courage and their determination to triumph over adversity are remarkable. Their ingenuity in finding simple, practical solutions to some of the problems presented by breast surgery and their delight in passing on their tips have been a pleasure to record. Their unselfishness in wanting to help other women in the same plight, even if only by holding out a hand and saying, 'it's all right, you can get through it,' has been inspiring. Certainly, they have convinced me that there truly is life after breast cancer. I hope that readers of this book will be equally persuaded.

Next I would like to thank the staff and Council members of the Breast Care and Mastectomy Association who have given me time and the benefit of their experience. A particular acknowledgement is due to Jacqueline Lee, Client Services Manager, whose technical knowledge about prostheses was invaluable to me.

I would like to thank Mr Dudley Sinnett, Mr Christopher Ward and Mr George Watts for their help and constructive comments on the chapters dealing with breast surgery and breast reconstruction.

I would like to acknowledge the enthusiasm and patience shown by my editor, Jane Graham-Maw. And last but by no means least, I wish to express my appreciation of David Bainton's tolerance and supportive understanding through the months of preparing and writing this book.

Carolyn Faulder, May 1992

# Foreword

**BY DR PATRICIA LAST**

There is no easy way to tell a woman that she has breast cancer. Yet each year surgeons, GPs, radiotherapists and specialists in chemotherapy have to face this task, separately and together. They often get it wrong, indeed it would be impossible to get it right every time.

Even if there were a perfect way to impart this intolerable news, few women would be able to appreciate it in the hurly-burly of the doctor's surgery.

Each year in the UK 25,000 women are told they have breast cancer. They need calm and privacy to come to terms with this evidence of their own potential mortality. And they need answers to their questions. These questions may be trivial or profound, and the answers must be there when they want them.

*Always A Woman* provides answers to a wide variety of questions. It gives the reader insight, the companionship of other women's experience, an authoritative approach to different treatments, and enables any woman to play an active part in her disease - if that is what she wishes. It also enables her to hand over her care completely to her doctors - if that is her choice.

Neither approach is necessarily better than the other, but a woman with breast cancer should be able to find out what her options are. This book gives her a handle on those options in a clear and friendly way - woman to woman.

Dr Patricia Last, FRCS FRCOG
Director, Women's Screening Unit, BUPA

# 1

## EARLY DAYS

'I'm sorry to have to tell you . . .' When someone starts a sentence like that you know you are about to hear bad news. If the place is a hospital and the person speaking is a doctor, and you have just been through some investigations for pain, or a lump or some other unusual change in your breast, your heart will lurch.

There is no easy way to tell someone that they have cancer. The doctor may be kind, the words carefully chosen, but nothing you hear is going to sound right to you. How could it, when what you are being told is that you have a disease which threatens your life? Even if you have been having suspicious symptoms, it will still come as a shock to have them confirmed.

You may feel yourself breaking out into a sweat, your mouth going dry, your breath coming out in shallow pants - all the signs of a panic attack. Or you may just feel terribly cold and stiff and remote. You may feel disembodied, as if you are floating above that person sitting on the edge of her chair who is listening so intently to what the doctor is telling her. She cannot be you. But of course she is.

# Can This Be Happening To Me?

We all react differently to bad news. And how we react is not
something over which we have any control. It doesn't really
matter. You may feel like crying or shouting with anger; you
may want to ask endless questions, or just curl up in a dark
room to think about it on your own; the important thing is
to get through this first painful ordeal - the passage from
ignorance to knowing the unpleasant truth - any way you can.
You will need all the help you can find. You may be surprised
by the reserves of strength that well up within you, but you
will also need the love and understanding of those who are
close to you as well as the support of the professionals caring
for you.

After the shock often comes denial.

*This can't be true. They've got it wrong. They can't be talking
about my tests, my body. There's been a mistake. It isn't me they
mean.*

Pell-mell, these thoughts hustle through your mind. In these
early days, when you are still trying to unravel the implications
of your bad news, it is normal to find yourself plunging wildly
on an emotional seesaw, occasionally taking respite from the
turbulence in a suspended state of disbelief. If you were
feeling perfectly well when you walked into the doctor's
surgery, it probably seems unthinkable that you could have
cancer. You may be finding it even harder to accept that
diagnosis if it results from a mammogram which has revealed
an impalpable cancer: that is to say, one which neither you
nor your doctor can feel merely by pressing with your fingers.

There are times when most of us prefer to deny a reality
for which we feel unprepared. This reaction is neither
cowardly nor unrealistic; rather, it should be seen as a natural
defence mechanism, a way of protecting ourselves from too
much pain until we have found a means of handling it. Most

people use denial as a temporary means of coping; a state of mind into which they can drop from time to time when their problems seem overwhelming. Then, when they feel a bit stronger, they can return to grappling with the here and now.

There will be some women, though, for whom denial is never an option. The bad news for them may almost come as a relief. They are the ones who may have been worried about their health for some time, but have been told by the doctor they consulted to go away because they have no cause for concern. Even today in the 1990s when cancer has ceased to be a taboo subject and we would hope that everyone is alert to danger signals it does still happen, unfortunately, that a woman can be given false reassurance. Sometimes even an experienced doctor may be mistaken in his preliminary examination and express himself too confidently, as happened with this woman at a London teaching hospital.

'My GP was sure it was just a blocked lymph duct after breastfeeding, and the consultant who aspirated what he called a cyst said that the fluid would be analysed, but it seemed fine. I went home and we opened a bottle of champagne to celebrate. A few days later I was telephoned by a doctor from the hospital who asked me to come to the next clinic. He wouldn't tell me why, though I spent half an hour trying to persuade him, and afterwards I rang up every day but nobody would tell me anything or put me through to the consultant. I felt very angry and deceived. That week was torture. Even at the clinic, where I had a new test, the consultant continued to be very reassuring, saying it was probably a cystic cancer. But it wasn't and it had already spread to the lymph nodes. One was affected and four were removed.'

*Vera*

Vera was 31 at the time, and the mother of two young children. She had always been haunted by the possibility of breast cancer because her own mother had died of it at a young age. Knowing she was in a high risk category, she had reported her lump promptly although she dreaded what might follow. Nine out of ten lumps will prove to be benign, so it is commendable for doctors to encourage women to be optimistic. They don't want to raise the alarm unnecessarily. Someone like Vera, however, who is well informed and has good reason to be worried, deserves to be taken seriously. Her questions should have been answered all along the line, and the doctors should have shared their doubts and taken her into their confidence. As it was, their prevarication, combined with a misconceived optimism, left her extremely angry when the truth finally emerged.

## Why Me?

This is a question we all ask ourselves when a disaster befalls us. Cancer produces this reaction in most people. And there really is no answer you can give. Very few forms of cancer have a direct cause-and-effect relationship. Smoking and lung cancer is an obvious exception, and there are some occupationally-induced cancers, but it is not so simple with breast cancer, as we will see in chapter two. There is nothing in a woman's circumstances or lifestyle at which she can point a self-accusing finger and say, 'if only I hadn't . . .'

This lack of an obvious target for blame doesn't remove the strong sense of guilt that so many women feel. If the cause is not physical then there must be some other reason, a woman will argue with herself, and start rummaging through her past life.

Have you caught yourself imagining you are being punished for some long-forgotten wrongdoing or even blaming yourself for having the 'wrong' personality? Too meek and submissive; not angry enough; not positive enough; aren't these supposed to be the cancer characteristics? In fact they are the glib comments we have probably all been guilty of making at some time or other, usually on no sounder basis than reading a couple of magazine articles on the psychology of cancer.

The truth is that cancer affects one in three of the population, and approximately 75 per cent of those cancers are estimated by the epidemiologists (doctors who study disease in populations) to be dietetically or environmentally induced. In other words the food we eat and the pollution in one form or other that we inflict upon ourselves and each other are the most common contributory factors. We can always change our diet, but if we don't know what causes the problem we can't be certain that we are achieving a significant improvement. Over the environment we probably have even less control, and over our personal birth package of genes and hormones, none at all.

Unfortunately, breast cancer is one of the cancers where an inherited predisposition - meaning you have close female relatives who developed the disease before the menopause - does put you at a considerably increased risk. If you think about it rationally, this can't be a cause for guilt. Your hormonal make-up doesn't dictate the sort of person you are, even if at times it makes you feel rotten. Rationality, however, has nothing to do with it. If a woman can't blame herself for being unlucky she may feel angry with her mother for putting her at risk, albeit unwittingly, or, if she has daughters, she may become consumed with guilt and desperately worried for their future wellbeing.

Apportioning blame may give you a temporary sense of achievement: you think at last you are finding some answers, but it soon wears off and you are likely to be left with an even stronger sense of failure. Down you plummet on your seesaw and hopelessness sets in. Why fight? Why bother with anything? you may ask yourself. You've been stricken with this disease and there's nothing you can do.

But there is. And so much of it is within your grasp, if only you can trust yourself to reach out for it. There are people to help you and there is much to learn, but it takes time to absorb a new reality. Some of this time will have to be spent on your own, as you start to take stock of your future. You can't escape your feelings, however good you may be at disguising them, and you have to live through them - distressing and painful as they are - before you will feel able to harness the energy they give you to good effect.

Anger, for instance, is a raw emotion which seizes many people by the throat at a time like this. It simply isn't fair, you say to yourself, and to others. You don't deserve this illness, you haven't done anything wrong and you are not ready for this - as if one ever is. In your frustration you may turn your wrath upon the people who have done the tests and told you the bad news. Now you give them a hard time. Kill the messenger. It's their fault. Deep down, you know this is being quite as irrational as feeling guilty, but it doesn't make your anger any easier to contain.

Anger is an uncomfortable state to be in. It makes you feel out of control; you tend to behave badly and then you feel worse because you have put yourself in a bad light. You may try to pretend you're not feeling angry, but this fools no-one and won't help you. All the same, anger has healing properties - it enables you to expel those negative thoughts which clog your will to move on and out of the impasse - so try, if you can, to clear the air by venting your feelings in a safe place with a safe person. Preferably it should be someone who is close to you and won't take what you say too personally but if this is not possible, a neutral third party could be just as good, someone like a counsellor, who has been trained to listen and is far too experienced to be shocked or upset by anything he or she hears.

Another way of dealing with strong emotions is to write a diary. It doesn't have to be done every day as a chore, but as the mood takes you. It's a marvellous way of talking yourself down. It also helps you to understand what is happening to you and even begin to see the way ahead, especially when you re-read it later in a calmer frame of mind.

On the whole, most people's anger is with the disease rather than with anyone in particular. There will be times, however, when you can't help feeling envious and bitter as you look around and wonder why others should have been spared when you have not been so fortunate.

'A woman in the bed next to me kept saying "Why me?" In the end I said to her: "Look, you're not alone. We're all in the same boat so why are you worrying?" That made her laugh and she said she felt better.'

*Una*

Una is a splendid matriarch, in her late fifties, who is already a great-grandmother. She has seen a lot of suffering and deprivation in her life, especially during the many years she worked in an American hospital for elderly black people, and she has experienced her own not inconsiderable share of personal adversity. Nonetheless she remains serene and cheerful. She takes a robust attitude to illness and to her breast cancer in particular, believing that there are always worse things that can happen to you, and she has seen some of them. 'Think lucky and you'll be lucky' is her philosophy.

# Who Can I Talk To?

Many women feel very lonely in these early days. This may
be because they are physically isolated; for instance, their
family has grown up and moved away, or they may be elderly,
or widowed, or just not know very many people. A woman
living on her own may be quite content with her single life
in normal circumstances, but this can change when she is
brought face to face with something serious like cancer. Even
if you are fortunate enough to be surrounded by a loving
family or have lots of good friends in whom to confide, and
enjoy a busy, interesting life, you may still feel overwhelmed
at times by a sense of isolation. There's no-one to talk to
because no-one can possibly understand what you are going
through. You have cancer. They don't.

'If only I could have talked to someone it would have
helped.'

*Isobel*

Isobel was 31 and married with two young daughters when
her first lump was discovered and a mastectomy was
performed. Three years later she had a nightmare in which
she dreamed a knife was being stuck into her other breast.
Waking up, she felt her breast frantically and found that a
lump had indeed appeared, literally overnight. Her GP
suggested she should come back two weeks later after his
holiday but she said 'to hell with that' and telephoned the
ward sister who had looked after her the first time. She was
treated as an emergency and a second mastectomy was
performed.

Isobel has no complaints about the medical care she was
given but even today, 15 years later, she still wonders why no-
one in the medical team – doctors and nurses alike – would
talk to her about what was really happening. Cancer was never

mentioned. As a young woman only recently transplanted from London to a remote rural area, she knew no-one outside the hospital to whom she could turn to or ask for advice. She was completely on her own except for her husband, who was unstinting in his support, but there were things Isobel guessed instinctively that only another woman who had been through a similar experience could help her with. Her unhappy isolation at that time explains why she is such an enthusiastic volunteer today for the Breast Care and Mastectomy Association. (See chapter ten for more about what volunteers do.)

In the last few years people have become much more willing to talk about cancer, but there are still far too many people being diagnosed who find they are expected to struggle with their problems in stoic silence. For the woman with breast cancer this unwelcome solitariness may start in the clinic from the moment when, the bad news delivered, the doctor leaves her alone to dress and find her own way home. Sometimes friends and acquaintances are not much more sympathetic. Some people actually turn away when they hear someone has cancer, or they fall ominously silent. Most cancer patients can tell you of at least one friend who has melted out of their life since their diagnosis.

There will be times, though, when it is you who longs to be left alone; you want to shut yourself away from all the kind offers of help and well-intentioned suggestions. All you seek is peace and quiet and time for reflection. Living through a crisis requires times for talking and times for silence, but it can be hard to persuade those who love you that you need sometimes to be on your own. They may feel rejected and show their hurt but if it matters to you, insist on it and try not to feel guilty. It is your life and your body, after all; only you can decide what your next steps are to be and how to take them.

'I feel very strongly that women should say what they want to say and be as they want to be. There was an expectation that you must be brave and that there's some way of being dignified about cancer, which I found very oppressive.'

*Vera*

These are just some of the emotions likely to engulf you in the early days after you have been given the bad news. Each woman reading this book will be going through her own private torment, so while you may identify with some of the situations described here, there may be others you have known more intensely. Fear, panic, despair, grief, horror, a tremendous sense of being lost and confused, are all feelings you are likely to experience. Try to go with them if you can, rather than resisting or denying them. Above all, it is important to acknowledge them and to allow yourself to admit that you feel terrible because once this has been expressed and is out in the open you will find it easier to put much of it behind you. Your unhappiness won't immediately dissolve or disappear; these feelings will recur many times, but because you recognize them you will feel stronger and more able to handle them.

## Picking Up The Pieces

When your emotions begin to subside you will start wondering what to do next. Most women realize immediately that they know very little about breast cancer. They may have read a few articles and they may even have been sufficiently aware of the implications of the disease to examine their breasts from time to time, but now they are faced with the reality they realize that they have everything to learn. Where can they find this information? Who will help them? What the doctor says tends to be forgotten almost as soon as it's heard, partly because of the stress but also because what he says is so unfamiliar.

This is the moment, if you are one of a lucky minority of patients, when you may have your first introduction to the breast care nurse counsellor. As her title suggests, she has been specially trained to care for women who have been diagnosed with breast cancer. In a well-organized set-up – usually a specially designated breast clinic in a major hospital – this nurse will be present when the news is first broken to you and she will stay with you throughout your subsequent treatment and check-ups, visiting you at home as well if necessary. She is someone to whom you can turn and of whom you can ask literally anything, in the sure knowledge that you won't be made to look foolish or ignorant. You can ask her all the big questions, as well as the small ones which you may have forgotten when you were with the doctor, or possibly you felt too shy to bring up because you were worried the doctor would see you as a time-wasting nuisance.

Unfortunately, most women will not be offered this opportunity of access to a kind and knowledgeable hospital 'friend'. Many are left to flounder in their misery, without anyone they can talk to freely, and unable even to lay their hands on a source of reliable information. Family and friends who want to help find that they are similarly frustrated; they too need help and information to support the one who is ill.

'I was so desperate I went to the telephone directory and looked up "cancer" but there was nothing under that entry that made me feel I could ring and ask my sort of questions.'
*Fern*

This is where this book comes in. As you will see from reading on, there is plenty of information and help available. It's just a matter of knowing where it is and how to make it work for you.

'From the time of hearing my diagnosis, it had seemed that my mind, emotions, social functioning and physical condition were pieces of a jigsaw spread out on a table in front of me. At first I had no means of starting to put the pieces together. Then slowly I began to think about moving one piece, then another. I decided to move my social functioning by talking openly to as many people as possible. I decided to move my psychological and emotional state [by giving myself time to feel my emotions].

My reward was that on the evening before surgery I felt I could reach out and begin to actually move the pieces. It was still going to take a long time to complete the jigsaw, but at least I had started.'

*Liz - cancer patient writing in BACUP News*, Spring 1989

Each woman is different. Our circumstances, our age, our personality, our experiences and our relationships all combine to create our own personal jigsaw of life. Although the individual pieces are uniquely shaped and ultimately form unique images, there remains enough common ground in an event like breast cancer for there to be value in sharing that experience. It helps you to define your own needs and discover ways of meeting them.

The following chapters aim to give you all the available information you need to unlock sources of help and support and thus enable you to put together again the pieces of your life. When the picture is complete, you may find, like the women quoted here, that life doesn't end with a diagnosis of breast cancer, though it certainly changes; sometimes it is actually renewed at a better, more satisfying level.

# 2

## TAKE YOUR TIME

Until recently it was regarded as good medical practice always to move very fast from the moment a breast cancer was suspected. Even though a GP might well have dawdled for months, playing down the fears of an anxious woman, perhaps suggesting she was being neurotic, once she entered the hospital it suddenly became a race against time. The surgeons believed it to be essential to remove the tumour as quickly as possible to prevent any further spread. This meant a woman would, quite routinely, be given the bad news one day and told to pack her bags and come into hospital for an operation the next. She would be given little or no time to discuss her situation, and the idea that she might wish to consider alternatives would not even be entertained.

The surgeon would not describe the procedures to her except in the barest outline, and no one would tell her what to expect afterwards. An inadequate consent form would be placed before her to sign, usually at the last moment, which required her to agree to a mastectomy (removal of the whole breast) if the malignancy was confirmed. This would be done by sending a 'frozen section' sample of the tumour down to the laboratory for an analysis lasting no more than ten minutes, while the anaesthetized patient and her surgeon waited in the operating theatre for the result. All but the most intrepid of women would sign the consent form obediently

and resign themselves to the expectation that they would
wake up without a breast. Most did, and had to learn to adapt
to their mutilation with little or no help from the medical
staff.

This is recent history. It was happening in hospitals all over
the UK even in 1990 but today, improved diagnostic methods
and more enlightened thinking should have made this
procedure redundant, except in those circumstances where
the patient herself asks her doctor to go ahead with a
mastectomy if it's immediately clear from the biopsy that she
has a cancer. Some women feel they don't want to go through
two operations in quick succession, and this is quite
understandable, but any woman who wants time to think it
over must be given it. Such extreme haste is seldom, if ever,
necessary and should not now ever happen against a patient's
will. Changes in the consent procedures protect the patient's
rights in this matter (see chapter four for more about giving
informed consent).

The truth is that although a diagnosis of cancer should
always be treated as a top priority, to delay a week, or even
longer, before commencing treatment is not going to make
a significant difference to the outcome except for those rare
cases where the tumour is growing visibly and rapidly. Most
breast lumps, by the time they are detected, whether with a
mammogram or by the woman or doctor feeling it, will have
been there for some time already. What matters now is that
the tumour be carefully examined, and that after all the
relevant tests have been carried out the woman is given as
much time as she needs to discuss her treatment options –
with her doctor and with her family.

Should you find yourself in a situation where you are finding
it difficult to resist the pressure being put on you to consent
to an immediate mastectomy, ask to see your doctor in the
company of your partner or a close friend or relative,

someone whom you can trust to support you and help you put the questions you want to ask. No woman should feel she is being pushed into making decisions about a matter of such vital importance to her before she feels confident she has all the information she needs.

'The waiting gave me time to let the news sink in and think about it. That was a good thing.'

*Katrina*

Katrina was 34 when her cancer was diagnosed and she, like Vera, felt that her worse nightmare had been realized, because she too had a mother who had died of breast cancer. She was fortunate in that she had a very understanding surgeon who sympathized with her and was prepared to give her all the time she needed. In fact, she waited a full month between the diagnosis and the operation; during that time, while she was having further tests, she joined a support group, went to relaxation classes and had some counselling.

'I was in a state of shock. I needed that time and I needed to talk. My way of coping is to talk a lot about whatever it is that's worrying me.'

*Katrina*

Not everyone feels as Katrina did. You may be one of those people who doesn't really care to know too much about their illness, so the last thing you want to do is talk about it. You may prefer to leave the decision-making to your medical advisors, taking the view perhaps that the doctors are the experts, so why not leave the responsibility for deciding about treatment entirely to them. Perhaps you feel that once the treatment is over you want to put the whole thing behind you and try to forget it ever happened. All this is very understandable and there's nothing wrong with such an attitude.

Everyone must feel free to try and handle their illness in the way that suits them best. Even so, don't rush. A few days more, if only to regain some kind of equilibrium after the shock, will give you time to think about your situation in more depth. Maybe there are one or two people close to you with whom you would like to talk things over because you believe they can give you good advice and help you approach the future in a calmer frame of mind. A short delay is not going to endanger your health.

## What Is Breast Cancer?

Unfortunately, there isn't a good answer to this question, by which I mean a clear definitive one; there is a mass of data surrounded by a lot of speculation. Why or how breast cancer occurs is still largely mysterious.

Although breast cancer has been a disease of women (and occasionally of men - one in 100 cases) since the dawn of history - the Egyptians, ancient Greeks and Romans all performed various forms of mastectomy - we still don't fully understand the natural history of the disease, let alone the best way of treating it. Cancer is a hugely variable disease. More than 200 different kinds can affect the various organs of the body and there are probably at least twenty variations of breast cancer alone, some of these having a better response to treatment than others. Like many other cancers, a malignancy in the breast usually shows itself as a lump of extra tissue which develops because the cells have gone on the rampage, dividing and sub-dividing in an uncontrolled way.

Some breast lumps grow rapidly; others may remain small and contained for a long time before making themselves apparent. For example, there is one called **ductal carcinoma**

**in situ (DCIS)** which grows in one or more of the milk ducts leading to the nipples. Only recently, with the development of X-ray techniques, has it been possible to detect this cancer at an early stage when it is very small (less than one centimetre) and is only visible on a mammogram as a microcalcification – a term for a minute abnormal cluster of cells. The problem for the doctors is deciding whether this does or does not betoken something more sinister. Many prefer to adopt a 'wait-and-see' policy, checking the woman at regular intervals to see whether there has been any change, and only intervening if there has. Even when this particular tumour is discovered at a later stage it is usually non-invasive; that means it won't have spread further into the breast or into other parts of the body. There may, however, be several of these microcalcifications dotted around in the same breast. In the past, these in-situ tumours were always removed by a mastectomy and the surgeon could honestly say the cancer had gone. Today, with the increased numbers of women having mammograms, more of these very early pre-cancerous conditions are being discovered; understandably, many surgeons feel reluctant about treating them with the drastic option of mastectomy. (For alternatives, now and in the future, see chapter three.)

First the good news.

The earlier a cancer is detected, the better the chances are of a cure. Women with early cancers who are treated promptly have a 30 per cent chance of cure and a very good long-term survival rate – 84 per cent will still be alive after five years. This is just another reason for making sure that if you are aged over 50, you go for the regular mammographic screen which you are entitled to have every three years. (This may change to two years if studies currently in progress show that more of the early cancers can be detected with shorter screening intervals).

Now the bad news.

Breast cancer is the major form of cancer among women in the United Kingdom, which has the highest incidence rate in the world. One in 12 women will develop it at some time in their life. The UK also has the worst death rate in the world - 28 per 100,000 women - and breast cancer is the major cause of premature death in women aged between 35 and 54.

Breast cancer in the UK accounts for:

26,000 new cases per year
16,000 deaths per year
5,000 deaths of women under the age of 65
One in five of all cancers among women.

These are terrible figures, and behind each one there is an individual woman whose life and happiness is threatened when she hears the diagnosis of breast cancer. She doesn't think of herself as a statistic, but as a human being with a life still to live; people she loves and who love her; things yet to do. Doctors tend to talk of 'survival' and 'mortality' in a somewhat detached way, but for the cancer patient these are grim realities which have suddenly been pushed into the forefront of their lives.

'I once heard a doctor talking about how women could hope to "survive" for perhaps two, five or ten years. That did make me angry. Surviving implies hanging on by one's fingertips. I decided I was going to *live* for 30 years at least.'

*Betty*

Betty Westgate founded the Mastectomy Association, now known as the Breast Care and Mastectomy Association (BCMA), in the early 1970s because she realized from her own experience of breast cancer (she had a mastectomy in 1968) how much women need to be able to confide in others who have 'been there' too. It's not that they are intrinsically different as a result of their illness, but it does cause many perfectly normal women to have emotional and practical problems which in those days were simply not recognized by the medical profession.

Betty's contempt for merely surviving has been well rewarded, for here she is all these years later, still in good health and still speaking out for the right of women with breast cancer to be regarded as complete human beings whose special needs should be met with compassion and understanding. Betty has never countenanced the idea that to lose a breast could somehow diminish you as a woman or in any way make you less worthwhile as a person; at the same time, she has always understood how women faced with this prospect might be feeling, because she too has suffered moments of desperation and anguish. Her example, and the work of the organization that she brought into being, demonstrate how important it is for us all to remember that there are real people behind the figures.

The statistics are chilling but they don't tell the whole story. Treatments have greatly improved in the last decade and there is now concrete evidence to show that women who are treated early enough really do improve their chances of living longer; even in those cases where the cancer eventually returns, it is more likely to be after a longer remission (disease-free interval) and the disease can usually be controlled more effectively (see chapter three).

## What Causes Breast Cancer?

Again this is one of those questions that can only be answered by a variety of speculative answers.

There is nothing that can be singled out as a definite cause, only a number of what are more accurately called 'risk factors', meaning that when one or more are present in a woman they appear to increase her likelihood of developing breast cancer. Many of these risk factors are related to her reproductive history: thus, an early menarche (first period); a late menopause; late childbearing (first child after the age of 30); and no children ever are all significant, and strongly suggest that there is a hormonal component (specifically oestrogen) in the development of many but not all breast cancers. Other significant risk factors are age (the older you are, the more at risk you become for any cancer), obesity and a history of benign breast lumps. On the plus side, breastfeeding and early childbearing are said to offer positive protection, but again there is no proof positive.

Then there is the family link. It is now well established that women who have one or more close female relatives from either side of the family – a mother, sister, cousin or aunt – who developed breast cancer before the menopause have a one in four chance of developing the disease themselves, often in their thirties. Recent research suggests that there is a faulty gene responsible for this familial variety of breast cancer, which accounts for about 10 per cent of all cases. The hunt is now on to find a genetic marker to track down the women who have inherited the susceptibility so that they can be screened regularly and, should it be appropriate, they may be offered some form of preventive treatment. The additional benefit of finding out who has inherited the gene (or possibly genes) means that those women who have not can be relieved of their anxiety for themselves, although their daughters will also need to be screened because they have a one in four chance of developing breast cancer. The ultimate aim of the medical researchers is to find something which will either repair the damaged gene or block its effects.

Other risk factors still being scrutinized include diet,

alcohol, stress, extended use of the contraceptive pill in young women before their first pregnancy, and prolonged use of hormone replacement therapy in older menopausal women. In various ways these are all related to lifestyle, which many women would feel encouraged to modify if the risk were definitely established. Possibly the most interesting one at the moment is diet. Many researchers believe that there is a definite causal link between a diet with too much fat and too little fibre and breast cancer. If this can be proved, it has been estimated that we could cut the annual UK breast cancer toll by half, saving at least 7,000 lives.

The evidence is convincing and more of it is coming in all the time. The theory is that too much fat in the diet creates an excess amount of oestrogen in the body. When this combines with a sluggish digestive system leading, as it often does, to constipation, the oestrogen is not eliminated. Maybe this explains why vegetarian women in Western countries have a lower incidence of breast cancer than their meat-eating sisters; so do Japanese and other Eastern women who live mainly on rice and vegetables. However, when they emigrate to North America and adopt the eating habits of the host population, they soon catch up; by the third generation they number as many cases of breast cancer, proportionate to their population, as their Western counterparts.

EPIC should provide us with the definitive answers. Recently launched, this is the appropriately-named European Prospective Investigation Into Cancer; it is the largest ever in-depth study to be set up with the purpose of looking specifically at the relationship between diet and cancer. Using the latest research techniques, it involves collecting detailed information about the eating habits and general health of more than 250,000 people in seven European countries who will then be followed up for at least 10 years to see who develops which cancer. (Approximately 4,000 cases would be

expected over this period in the UK sample of 85,000).
However, as early as 1997, which marks the first five years,
the researchers are confident they will already have
discovered some strong pointers about dietary factors – those
that promote cancer as well as those with a positive protect-
ive effect – particularly in relation to the bowel and
breast cancers which are major killers in the developed
world.

However, while we wait for this information, and
irrespective of whether or not we have cancer, it does no harm
to reconsider our diet. Adequate portions of fresh fruit and
vegetables every day will ensure we get the vitamins and fibre
we need; we will also be doing our hearts a good turn by
reducing our fat intake.

Stress may also play a part in some cases of breast cancer.
It certainly can't always be coincidence that a cancer often
develops in someone who has suffered a traumatic experience
or has been through a long period of prolonged stress. A loss
of some kind can be a typical harbinger – a bereavement,
going through a divorce, or losing a job are all major life
events – but to say that stress causes cancer may be too crude.
It is more probable that the stress acts as a trigger, probably
by depressing the immune system, thus debilitating the body
and making it incapable of fighting off attack from hostile
agents. Although we still understand so little about the
mind/body interaction, we do know enough by now to realize
that the one cannot be considered, or treated, in isolation
from the other. The holistic approach to healing is all-
important, especially in the treatment of a disease where
complete cure is not always certain. The complementary
therapies play a part in that healing process, sometimes in a
major way and sometimes simply by sustaining the patient
through the rigours of the orthodox therapies (see chapters
four and seven).

# What Happens Now?

Before your doctor can decide what treatment he or she thinks is most appropriate for your condition, it will be necessary to do some further tests. If it was you or your partner who found the lump, all you will probably have had so far is a clinical examination backed up by a mammogram. However, if you are aged between 50 and 65 and have taken advantage of the national breast screening programme, the first inkling that something might be wrong could have resulted from the doctor seeing a suspicious outline on the mammogram. In all cases, a mammogram which gives cause for concern should be followed up by a biopsy, because no sensible doctor wants to commit him- or herself to a diagnosis of cancer without being absolutely sure that it is indeed present.

The biopsy can either be done as a fine needle aspiration in the out-patient clinic or as an excision under general anaesthetic. The first way (fine needle biopsy) is a relatively quick and painless procedure, and involves removing a few cells only from the lump with a needle and syringe. The second method may mean staying overnight in hospital, because the whole lump is removed under general anaesthetic. Whichever method is used, the suspect tissue is sent to the pathology laboratory for careful analysis. The pathologist's report will guide the doctor (or doctors, because very often breast cancer is treated by a medical team incorporating complementary specialisms) in selecting a treatment programme.

Almost the first, most important question they need to resolve is what stage the cancer is at. Unfortunately this is not as simple as it might appear because, although examining the tumour tissue will give the doctor a good idea of the type of cancer, it may not indicate whether it is early or late. Size is not always a trustworthy indication of the stage.

As an approximate guide, there are four stages of breast cancer, but within these stages there are many individual variations which can prove quite deceptive. Early breast cancer (stage I) is when the tumour, usually very small, is confined to the breast alone. Stage II is still defined as early breast cancer, but it means it has spread into one or more of the lymph nodes under the arm on the same side as the affected breast. Stage III indicates more advanced breast cancer. The tumour will be quite large, perhaps as much as five centimetres, and it may well be attached to the muscle of the chest wall. Stage IV means that the cancer is advanced and has spread to other parts of the body causing secondary cancer, whether or not the primary tumour in the breast is large or small.

Before proceeding to surgery or other treatment for the tumour, there are several tests which doctors will carry out if they think there is any likelihood of spread. They may do these tests even if they think it's most unlikely that the cancer has progressed beyond the breast, simply because they want to be as sure as they can be that they have all the information they need before they proceed. These tests are likely to include scans of your bones, your lungs and your liver. None of them is painful - they involve injecting a vein with a radioactive substance which will be picked up by a scanner if it moves to an abnormal (i.e. cancerous) area in any of these sites.

Of course, such tests are going to cause you concern, but try to see them as a form of insurance rather than as an indication that the worst has already happened. If your doctors can eliminate the possibility of spread, they will be able to offer you a more moderate course of treatment as well as a good deal more hope for the future.

# 3

## A NEW AGENDA

### Yesterday

Until the 1970s there had been virtually no change in the treatment of breast cancer for almost a century, apart from some relatively minor modifications in surgical techniques and some limited experimentation with hormonal therapy. The mastectomy was the operation of choice, usually followed by a six-week course of radiotherapy to mop up any latent cancer cells in the breast and armpit area. Younger women who were still menstruating might also have their ovaries removed, thereby inducing an early artificial menopause. This operation was done because it had been known since the late nineteenth century that, in some women at least, breast cancer appeared to be oestrogen dependent; the mechanism of this connection was not understood.

The first real signal for change came when a few doctors, questioning their own complacency, began to examine the figures more closely. Why weren't the rates for cure, long-term survival and mortality getting better? Could they (the doctors) be doing too much? Amputating breasts might not, after all, be the life-saving operation they had always thought it to be. Or were they doing too little? Should they be offering other treatments to women in addition to, or instead of, surgery and radiotherapy, such as the drugs which were now being used for some other cancers? If so, which ones?

These important medical debates gained in urgency as women increased in assertiveness, especially those who were influenced by the rekindled women's movement in the late sixties. An essential element of the new wave of thinking among these women was an interest in health issues, particularly those which concerned their demand to be more in control - of their lives and, therefore, of their bodies. It was no longer a case of the occasional stroppy woman who was either asking for an alternative to mastectomy or downright refusing it who would then, for her pains, be branded as 'difficult' in her medical records. Women in general were becoming less compliant about the treatments being offered to them, and more openly intolerant of the medical profession's time-honoured paternalistic attitude towards patients - of both sexes, it has to be said. Where women led, the media, ever alert to the possibilities of a tasty 'human interest' story, followed.

By the mid-1980s, breast cancer had ceased to be a taboo subject. This meant that women could openly express their discontent without fear of being stigmatized, and those doctors who were more concerned about their patients than their prestige could feel free to utter the brutal truth aloud: medicine had got nowhere with this killer disease. The time had come for a radical rethink about every aspect of the management of breast cancer. To be fair, there were individuals in various branches of health care - psychologists, social scientists and nurses as well as doctors - who had already started down the road of reappraisal, but it was now well recognized that any new strategies would have to be buttressed by sound research. That meant setting up carefully-planned clinical trials to compare different treatments; enrolling large cohorts of patients, because numbers are essential when seeking to establish a difference significant enough to warrant a change of practice; and finally, monitoring the progress of the trials with rigour and analysing the results equally scrupulously.

Research of this calibre can't be done in a hurry and many trials had to be repeated, sometimes for good scientific reasons, the most obvious being the need to be certain it wasn't a one-off fluke, but quite often because there was a legitimate doubt about the validity of the results. Perhaps the original protocol was flawed; or the conduct of the trial itself was suspect; or, and this can happen very easily, despite the claims of scientists to have a better handle on objective truth than most of us, bias had crept into the interpretation of the results.

Many lessons were learned along the way, including one which has caused bitterness and controversy and is not yet wholly resolved; this is that human beings have an autonomy which must be respected even when, as patients, they become sick and vulnerable. This means you can't treat them like laboratory rats or grade them like peas, even if you are quite convinced that what you are doing is for their own good. Doctors are learning slowly that patients' feelings must be considered, and their values, often quite different from those of their carers, always respected. Above all, their informed consent has to be sought and willingly given before they are entered into a trial. The science may be first rate but, if it's not supported by generally accepted moral principles like telling the truth, it offers no guarantee of good ethical practice. To achieve results by deception is an unworthy way to make progress.

## Today

I have thought it worth briefly recounting this recent history of changing attitudes and practice in the treatment of breast cancer because it forms the backcloth against which the promising new agenda for action in the nineties has been drawn up. Already there is much more choice; furthermore, the options that can be offered to a woman today tend to be based on firmer scientific ground than in the past, when it was the doctor who made the decision, guided by his or her clinical judgement and experience, and usually without any discussion with the woman to find out what her personal feelings might be. Being asked to make choices can, however, present its own difficulties. For one thing, it implies a willingness to take responsibility for your decisions in an area where you may have little or no previous experience. (See chapter four for more discussion about choice.)

You should also remember that breast cancer is very variable and each woman diagnosed with it will present a slightly different picture to her doctor. Quite apart from the type and stage of the cancer, the doctor will have to take into account personal factors like her age, her family status, her social circumstances and her previous medical history. That is why so often two women lying in bed next to each other in the hospital ward, seemingly both with the same stage of disease, will find they have had different treatments. Another possible reason is that they are under different doctors, each of whom has a strong preference for a particular, different treatment.

Or it may be that you are being treated in a hospital which has a cancer centre. (At the time of writing there are 54 such centres throughout the UK, not enough to serve a population where one in three people has a lifetime chance of developing cancer but, hopefully, there will be many more by the end of the century). Here your treatment will be planned by a team of doctors who are all cancer specialists in their own branch of medicine and who will go to some lengths to discuss every step carefully with you. The core members of an oncology team (oncology is the branch of medicine dealing with the study and treatment of cancer) comprise a physician, radiotherapist, surgeon and breast care nurse, and they will be assisted by others who also have special skills for looking after cancer patients.

## Treatments

### SURGERY

For most women this is still the most usual first line treatment for early breast cancer. There are two main types of operation: mastectomy and lumpectomy.

A **mastectomy** involves either removing the whole breast (total) or a good portion of it (partial). There are various

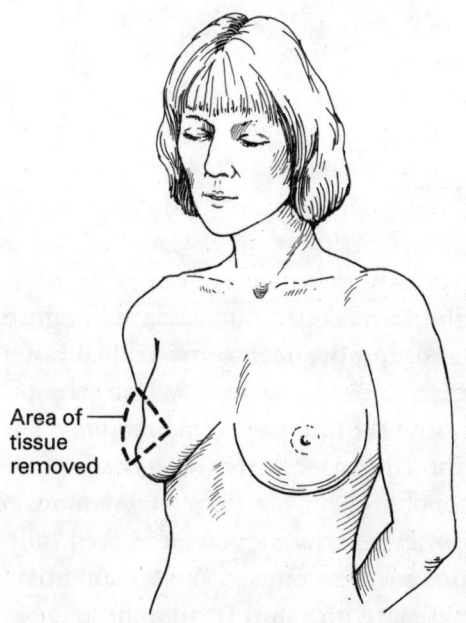

Area of
tissue
removed

*Fig 1 Segmentectomy (also known as tylectomy or quadrantectomy).*
*Up to a quarter of breast tissue may be removed together with the lump.*

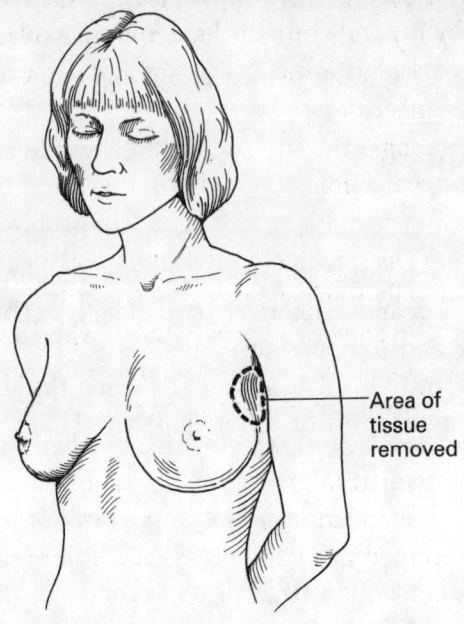

Area of
tissue
removed

**Fig 2 Lumpectomy.**
*Only the lump is removed, together with a small amount of surrounding tissue.*

names for the latter operation such as **segmentectomy**, **tylectomy** and **quadrantectomy**. It really depends how much tissue is removed and from which part of the breast, but whichever one it is, a partial mastectomy is always more extensive than a **lumpectomy**.

A lumpectomy, as the name suggests, is a more conservative (reduced) operation. The surgeon removes only the lump, together with a small amount of surrounding tissue, the least that is compatible with safety. It's important, obviously, not to leave behind any cancer cells but there is, nonetheless, a somewhat greater risk of what is called local recurrence with a lumpectomy. This means a return of the cancer to the site of the scar but, should this happen, it can usually be removed easily and rapidly with a further short course of radiotherapy. Sometimes, though, it proves resistant and a mastectomy may ultimately be necessary.

As regards long-term survival, it has now been definitely proved in several clinical trials that there is no difference between having a mastectomy or a lumpectomy for early breast cancer. This medical certainty is reassuring for those women who really don't want to lose their breast. However, there are cases, even with an early cancer, when a mastectomy is either unavoidable or may be preferable for reasons which could be medical, cosmetic or personal.

Medical reasons include the following: when there is more than one primary tumour in the breast or several areas of suspect microcalcification, or when the tumour is either very large, or positioned in such a way that it's impossible for the surgeon to remove it without taking much of the breast at the same time. Typically, this happens when it is directly behind the nipple. On cosmetic/aesthetic grounds, a woman with small breasts may decide that even though the lump is small, a lumpectomy will still cause her quite serious disfigurement; she finds it preferable to have a mastectomy backed up by the option, should she want it, of a breast reconstruction (see chapter nine). Personal reasons are as individual as each woman, but a very usual one is that no matter how reassuring the doctor may be about her prospects, the woman herself knows she will feel happier and more secure about her future if she has the whole breast removed.

'I wanted it all out. I wanted to feel sure it had gone. I reckoned it was better for my children to have a one-breasted mother than no mother'.

*Jean*

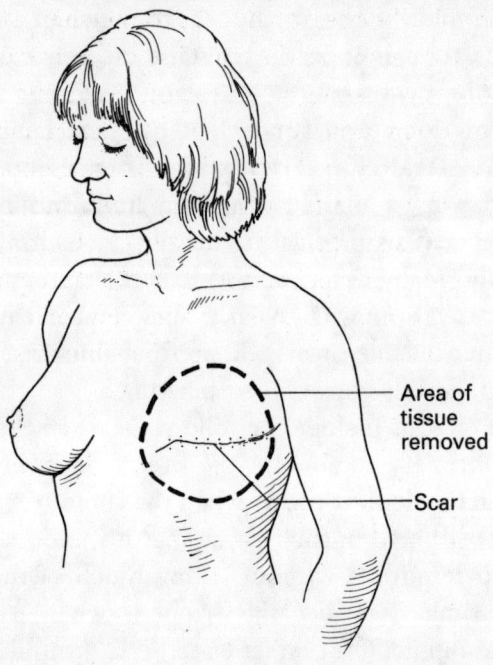

Area of
tissue
removed

Scar

**Fig 3  Simple mastectomy.**
*Breast tissue only removed.*

The usual total mastectomy involves removing all the breast
tissue including the nipple, leaving a thin straight scar across
the chest. This is called a **simple** mastectomy. An alternative
to this is the **subcutaneous** mastectomy which leaves the
skin and nipple intact by removing the breast tissue through
an incision made under the breast, and it is particularly
favoured by doctors who are offering reconstruction at the
same time.

There are, however, times when a doctor will need to do
a more extensive operation, called a **modified radical**
(sometimes known as a **Patey** after the surgeon who invented

it). This may be necessary, for instance, if the cancer has spread beyond the breast tissue on to the chest wall, in which case it can no longer be described as an early cancer, but the doctor may have some other reason for doing it. Never be afraid to ask why a particular type of operation or treatment is being offered to you. The modified radical entails removing all the breast tissue and the axillary lymph nodes (see below for more explanation). Additionally, it includes removing some muscle - the pectoralis minor - and possibly some internal lymph nodes as well if they appear to be affected. The scar will be longer and probably thicker.

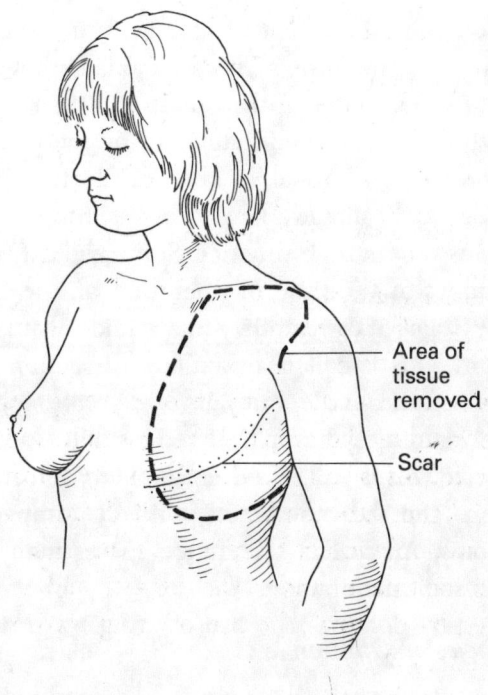

**Fig 4 Modified radical or Patey mastectomy.**
*Breast tissue and some underlying chest muscle removed.*

With all these mastectomies reconstruction is possible, either immediately or at a later date. As we said earlier, it's very important to establish whether there has been any spread of the cancer beyond the breast, because this will help the doctors to plan your total treatment following surgery. The minute cancer cells (called **micrometastases**) which may break off from the primary tumour, and travel in the bloodstream and lymphatic system to seed themselves in distant sites in the body, are difficult to spot, even with scans.

A useful check which surgeons have been doing for a long time is to examine the lymph nodes in the axillary glands, under the arm, by doing a lymphadectomy. These glands, like similar ones all over the body, act as watchdogs, always on the lookout for the threat of attack from disease and ready to fight it. In the case of breast cancer, they serve as the immune barrier between the breast and the rest of the body. If they show signs of being affected by the primary tumour in the breast it is probable, but not always inevitable, that cancer cells will already have crossed into the body.

Surgeons vary in their practice. Some will extract only a few lymph nodes at the time of operating on the breast and, if there is no sign of cancer, they may decide against any further treatment. This is called an axillary dissection or sampling. Others prefer to take out all 30 lymph nodes to make absolutely sure they haven't missed a single one which might be affected. This is called an axillary clearance. Either operation can be combined with a lumpectomy or a mastectomy. An axillary clearance spares many women the need for radiotherapy.

## Differences of Opinion

### How Many Lymph Nodes?
Surgery has always been subject to fashion, and the treatment of breast cancer is no exception. The welcome trend in favour

of reducing the number of mastectomies has also included cutting down on the number of lymphadectomies. Doctors have either not been doing them, if they are confident the cancer is very early, or they have confined themselves to taking a limited sample, perhaps no more than four to six nodes, for testing.

Some surgeons are now cautioning against this practice because they believe that it is putting women at needless risk not to make a complete node inventory. Their arguments are convincing, and are based on the established fact that the likelihood of relapse in breast cancer is directly related to the number of lymph nodes that show metastases (cancer spread). Therefore, say these doctors, it is advisable to remove all the nodes and not run the risk of missing some that are cancerous. They also point out that since adjuvant chemotherapy is now known to improve the prospects in particular of pre-menopausal women (see page 53), it is very important to have a precise picture of their lymph node status before prescribing the regimen. Another advantage of an axillary clearance is that it gives all women of any age at least as good a chance as radiotherapy - and these surgeons maintain that it is a considerably better one - of not getting a local recurrence. Finally, it also seems that the chance of getting lymphoedema - a swollen arm caused by trapped lymph fluid which can become a troublesome chronic condition - is much less (5 per cent as compared with something over 50 per cent) if the armpit area is treated surgically rather than with radiotherapy.

## Timing of Surgery

Some doctors believe that pre-menopausal women should have their operation 12 or more days after their last menstrual period. This view is based on recent research at Guy's Hospital in London, where analysis of the records of women who had surgery for breast cancer between 1975 and 1985 showed that there was a significant survival advantage for the women who had their surgery in the second half of their menstrual cycle - 84 per cent were alive after 10 years as compared to 54 per cent for those who had their operation between 3 and 12 days after their period. The theory is that this is because more oestrogen circulates in the first half of the menstrual cycle when it's unopposed by progesterone, the other female hormone whose level rises later in the cycle to counteract some of the effects of oestrogen. If this proves correct, the doctors at Guy's estimate that judiciously timed surgery could possibly save up to 600 lives a year. (About 6,000 pre-menopausal women are diagnosed with breast cancer in the UK each year.)

Doctors tend to snarl and pick over each other's research results like dogs over bones. This particular theory is exciting a lot of debate at the moment and other hospitals are now running their own reviews of patient records. Some have already disputed the Guy's team's findings but since hospital records are kept according to different systems, and perhaps not all of them with such meticulous care, it may be some time before we get a firm answer. Meanwhile, my advice to any woman under the age of 50 who has not yet had her menopause is to play safe and insist on having her operation in the second half of her cycle.

## RADIOTHERAPY

This is a treatment which can be used on its own to eradicate a tumour but more commonly, at least in the UK and the United States, it is used as a follow-up to surgery. It has been a standard treatment for all forms of cancer ever since the early years of this century when it was discovered that irradiation could destroy cancer cells completely and for ever. Cancer cells, once irradiated, can't regenerate themselves, unlike healthy cell tissue which can recover from a certain amount of damage. For many years, radiotherapy was the only other treatment, apart from surgery, which was available to a breast cancer patient.

It works by directing high energy rays on to carefully pinpointed areas in the breast and armpit where the doctor thinks there might be stray cancer cells which escaped the surgeon's knife. Radiotherapy is essentially what is called a local treatment: it focuses on the tumour site and surrounding area with the aim of preventing recurrence, or at least considerably reducing the risk, but it can't deal with cancer cells that may have already escaped into the body.

There are basically two ways of giving radiotherapy:

1) by beaming either gamma rays or x-rays on to the treatment area. This procedure requires careful planning, including the use of a simulator so that the radiographer can rehearse the actual treatment as it will be given to you. The treatment itself, delivered either by a Cobalt machine (gamma rays), or a Linear Accelerator (x-rays), takes only a few minutes, but it usually extends over a period of four to six weeks, five days a week. The choice of machine depends largely on the size and shape of your breast and what is available in the unit.

2) by placing radioactive iridium wires in the breast after the lump has been removed. This is called an interstitial implant and some surgeons are now implanting these wires immediately after removing the lump, during the same operation. The wires are connected to a machine for approximately six hours a day, and radiation is then administered in a constant dose to the tumour site. The advantage of this treatment is that although you have to stay in hospital for it, it lasts no longer than three to five days. Then the wires are removed, the treatment is over and you can go home and hope to put it behind you.

## Other Uses of Radiotherapy

### Sole Form of Treatment

Sometimes a tumour is so invasive and growing so rapidly that doctors feel it is safer to irradiate it rather than excise it surgically.

French doctors have another reason for choosing radiotherapy rather than surgery as a first line treatment. French women have always firmly resisted the idea of accepting a mastectomy unless it is absolutely unavoidable, so for many years, their doctors, sympathetic to this point of view, have been offering them radiotherapy alone, with very good results.

Radiotherapy techniques are much more refined and accurate than they were, and so is the technology which delivers the dosage. Even so, treatment varies quite considerably, in part because of who is doing it but also because each woman presents as an individual with a particular sort of tumour in a breast of a particular size and shape.

The breast which has been treated by radiotherapy alone often continues to look much as it always did, but sometimes there is a delayed reaction and it begins to shrink a bit and perhaps harden. It may become discoloured and in some cases become quite deformed. Occasionally, despite the radiotherapy, the cancer recurs in the same breast, in which case a mastectomy will be necessary. Although these are not very likely occurrences, it's important that women should be aware of the possibility. Knowing what could happen may influence their choice of treatment.

### Palliative

Radiotherapy can be an effective painkiller should the cancer recur, particularly when the secondaries are in the bones.

## ADJUVANT THERAPIES

These are treatments which are prescribed in addition to surgery and radiotherapy. They are the following:

**Chemotherapy** – a combination of cytotoxic (anti-cancer) drugs used in various permutations to kill any stray, undetected cancer cells which may have escaped into the body. It is usually, but not exclusively, given to pre-menopausal women under the age of 50.

**Hormone therapy** is usually either chemical or surgical. In its chemical form it is either a synthetic hormonal compound which works as an anti-oestrogen or a form of anti-adrenal treatment. Commonly known as tamoxifen, it is taken as a tablet and can also be prescribed under the names of Novaldex, Tamofen and Noltam. It is usually given to post-menopausal women over the age of 50, but it can also be given to younger women. It can be used with good results as the sole treatment for frail elderly women whom the doctor would like to spare from surgery.

**Ovarian ablation** (the alternative form of hormone therapy) is the removal of the ovaries either by surgery or irradiation, thus producing an artificial menopause. As a therapy it has been in existence for more than a century but it has recently fallen out of fashion in favour of chemotherapy which can, as a side effect, also produce a permanent cessation of menstruation. The reasoning is obvious: if breast cancer is oestrogen-dependent it's important to remove any stimulus, and the ovaries are the main source of oestrogen during a woman's reproductive years. In view of recent unexpected findings (see below), ovarian ablation could well become popular once more.

Until recently, all these treatments were regarded by many doctors as optional extras. (For a fuller explanation of how they work, how they are given and their side effects see chapter seven). Their use depended either on the personal view of a doctor who favoured them as a form of extra insurance against recurrence, or, more scientifically, because the doctor believed the evidence in favour of a particular treatment to be good but that it needed to be proved. Therefore, he or she would enter patients into a trial where treatments were compared on a randomized allocation.

These trials have been going on since the 1970s and, as encouraging results started to come through, a growing number of doctors became convinced that adjuvant therapy should be regarded as an essential, rather than optional, element in the treatment of early breast cancer. What also began to emerge was that there was a clear distinction in treatment response between older and younger women; with 50 as the breakpoint age. Women over that age appeared to do particularly well on tamoxifen, whereas the younger, pre-menopausal women fared better on chemotherapy.

The publication of two landmark papers in the *Lancet* in January 1992 confirmed medical optimism and signposted new directions for the future both in treatment and research. The findings are based on a worldwide collaborative overview of 133 randomized trials involving 75,000 women, all being treated for early breast cancer – stage I and stage II (see page 34 for definitions). It is a remarkable study and the results are impressive. It is also good to note that the authors of the report give due credit to the women involved. Certainly, were it not for their participation, this information, with its valuable implications for the treatment of future patients, would not now be available. It's to be hoped that they were all fully aware and consenting participants in their trials.

Here is a summary of these important findings. Women of all ages in these two categories who receive one or more of these adjuvant therapies have a significant survival benefit over 10 years. It was already known that both hormonal therapy and ovarian ablation showed a modest improvement over five years. This study shows that the improvement becomes even more marked over 10 years. For every million such women, these benefits could mean 100,000 extra survivors over 10 years or 10,000 more women alive worldwide each year. In Britain it has been estimated that a staggering 1,000 extra lives could be saved every year by the judicious application of these adjuvant therapies.

Further research is now necessary to work out much more precisely the best type of therapy, (or combination of therapies), the dosage and its duration for women who have particular tumours in particular age groups. Table 1 gives an overall indication of the respective benefits of each treatment in various age groups.

---

## WHAT EVERY PATIENT AND DOCTOR SHOULD KNOW

Cancer specialists now feel confident the new study results give them more 'certainty' in advising on treatment options. The chart overleaf shows the numbers of extra 10-year survivors per 100 middle-aged women who receive different treatments following surgery for breast cancer which has spread to several lymph nodes.

Women whose cancer has not spread are less at risk: four in five may expect to remain trouble free so their absolute benefit from additional treatment is placed at around 12 for every 200 treated. Eighty per cent of all breast cancer patients are aged 50 or more.

| Treatment | Extra Lives Saved (per 100 over 10 years) |
|---|---|

## Age over 50:

**Tamoxifen alone for two years (specialists believe longer treatment may have more effect)**     **8**

This drug appears to act by blocking natural supplies of oestrogen which may, in some women, fuel cancer spread. The benefits in delaying cancer recurrence in the same or other breast are the same whatever the starting age or stage of disease.

**Multiple therapy with powerful cancer cell killing drugs alone**     **5**

Usually given for six months or more, though the good news is that shorter courses can be as effective.

**Tamoxifen plus chemotherapy**     **12**

Although chemotherapy is generally less effective among older women, this striking combined effect could lead some specialists to rethink their approach.

## Age under 50:

**Introduction of artificial menopause (ovarian ablation) through surgery or irradiation alone**     **11**

The striking new results for this way of blocking the body's supply of oestrogen hormone could lead to the resurgence of a method which has dropped out of fashion.

**Multiple therapy with cancer cell killing
drugs alone**                                                          **10**

**Artificial menopause plus chemotherapy**               **12**
It is not clear if the two together offer a definite
advantage as at least some of the effects of
chemotherapy lie in stopping periods and
blocking oestrogen supplies.

*Source: ICRF's Cancer Studies Unit, Oxford*

---

# Tomorrow

There are exciting new treatments in the pipeline but it will
be some time yet, several years undoubtedly, before they have
been tested sufficiently to ensure their safe use as routine
treatment for breast cancer.

**Laser therapy** plays an important part in the development
of 'keyhole' surgery, so-called because of the minute incisions
it requires and the much reduced recovery time that follows,
compared with traditional surgery. It is already being used for
a variety of conditions, most of which are not life-threatening
but can be seriously disabling, like gallstones or a damaged
spinal disc.

The beauty of laser therapy is that it is swift, precise and
minimally invasive. To explain it in very broad terms, it is a
form of microsurgery which operates by inserting
miniaturized cameras and telescopes attached to instruments
through tiny holes surrounding the area to be treated. Images
of the target are thrown up on a screen, enabling the surgeon
to direct the instrument from outside the body to destroy the
targeted tissue. Doctors are excited by this new surgery
because it is elegant, safe and effective as well as being far
less traumatic for the patient. Their patients like it for the

same reasons, and particularly appreciate that they are left with no scars and can return to normal life so much more quickly. Hospital managers are keen on it because it is cost-effective and enables them to speed up their patient throughput, at the same time freeing beds for those cases where treatments must be followed by a period of hospital nursing. Most laser operations can be done on an out-patient day-surgery basis, even when it's necessary to use a general anaesthetic.

Now there is a team at the National Medical Laser Centre, located at University College Hospital in London, which is experimenting with new techniques to remove malignant tumours. They are especially interested in those found in the liver, pancreas and breast, all large solid organs which allow the doctor plenty of room to focus on to the tumour, using extremely sophisticated imaging technology to pinpoint its precise position. Various refinements of laser therapy are being tried in a small pilot study. One for which the doctors have high hopes involves threading a flexible laser fibre into a fine needle which is then inserted into the breast at the precisely targeted point. The powerful laser beams are directed on to the tumour and 'cook' it (thermal coagulation is the technical term) until all the cells are killed. The dead tumour tissue is left in the breast to be absorbed by the body's natural healing mechanism. This procedure lasts less than 15 minutes and requires only a local anaesthetic. It leaves no scarring at all.

> 'It was not unpleasant or painful, but I did feel immense heat for about 10 minutes. It was a bit like having sunburn under my skin, right inside my breast'.
>
> *Rosemary, Sunday Times*, 24th November 1991

At the time of writing, only women who are already scheduled for a mastectomy are taking part in the trial. Their participation is an unselfish one, because they all understand that the treatment is entirely experimental at this stage and can't benefit them. As soon as the doctors feel happy with the technique and know what effects it produces, they hope to set up a clinical trial comparing laser therapy either combined with tamoxifen or on its own. If that is successful there will be many other combinations to try out. The doctors developing it anticipate that it will be especially welcome to women who may have a very small early cancer in the breast, for instance, DCIS, which is only visible on a mammogram.

Success will mean not only a major treatment breakthrough but, hopefully, will encourage many more women to come forward early and not to refuse their screening invitation. Fear of mutilation haunts many women and makes some of them delay far too long in seeking medical advice.

**Gene therapy** is something to look forward to in the next century. It may well render all the treatments in use today obsolete, but although fascinating and very promising theories abound, including several reports of scientific discoveries relating to breast cancer genes, it is still going to be some time before the research will have reached a stage where it can be taken forward into treatment applications.

**Active specific immuno therapy** which involves using the body's own immune system to attack and destroy cancer cells is another pioneering development. A pilot study at Guy's Hospital investigating patients' responses to a particular mucin molecule which changes in breast cancer could be the first step down the road to producing a vaccine against breast cancer.

# 4

## CHOICES AND DECISIONS

### Making An Informed Choice

No-one would choose to be diagnosed with cancer. That's obvious, but when it happens and you feel as if you have been plunged into a nightmare from which you can't awaken, it may seem as if you are losing control of every part of your life. The disease takes you over. Other people are in charge of your destiny - doctors, nurses, paramedics - you have become part of their daily work, a new name on their list. They examine you attentively, deal with you professionally, and - hopefully - with kindness, but, at the end of the day when their work is finished, they can go home and forget you. Meanwhile, where has the real 'you' gone? You feel passive, like a child who waits to be told what to do, unable to take any initiative because you have no experience and no knowledge of what is happening to you.

You are told the facts - the diagnosis and possibly the prognosis. You are told the treatment you should have. Your questions are answered, sometimes patiently and at great length; sometimes, alas, hurriedly and with little sympathy. You feel yourself to be a different person. You have been transported to another world, your needs and priorities have changed and you are looking desperately for familiar signposts, something to tell you how to behave in this new situation. The hospital where you now seem to spend so much time having tests and discussing treatments is an alien environment, yet it is one into which you find yourself sinking almost with relief. It's fast becoming a refuge from the 'real world' outside with all its demands and hustling impatience with any weakness. This unnerves you and you begin to wonder if you are becoming institutionalized.

And now new burdens appear. Quite apart from trying to cope with your own emotions after the diagnosis, a situation we have already explored earlier in this book, other people may be unloading their problems on to you. Some of these may be a knock-on effect of your illness, for instance, people close to you who are finding it hard to accept that you are seriously ill. Other problems may be quite distant from your own, but you find your vulnerability exposes you to people who want to share their pain and hurt with someone they may not even know very well, but who they sense will understand their difficulties because they have been similarly wounded. Sometimes you may want to do the same.

Some of this emotional upheaval is helpful, some is not. It may be difficult to handle, especially when it involves people you care for and whose feelings you don't want to hurt. Sometimes you are going to have to say, quite firmly, 'Look, just shut up for a bit and listen to me. I'm the one who's got cancer. I'm the one who needs help.' And, as time goes on, you will be looking for that help from all quarters.

'Take your time. Write down your questions. Talk openly about your cancer to your family and friends. Talk to other patients. Seek as much support as you can. Be very kind to yourself. Delegate work. Let others do the washing-up, the ironing, the cooking. You've got to do the thinking and the planning. You need the time to yourself.'

*Angela, Woman's Hour*, BBC Radio 4, January 1992

The first thing you have to decide for yourself is how much you want to know. And, following on from that, whether you want to be involved in making decisions about your treatment. Some people genuinely would prefer to know as little as possible about their illness. They find it upsetting to be asked whether they have preferences for a particular treatment, lumpectomy, say, instead of mastectomy, or radiotherapy as well as chemotherapy. It worries them to think that a doctor could possibly admit to being uncertain whether one treatment is better than another. They want to feel that the doctor is the expert who knows all there is to know about the disease, and that they can safely deliver themselves into his or her competent hands.

Those who complain that too many doctors think they are God should ask themselves why this is such a common phenomenon. Perhaps it's because we need to turn them into someone all-powerful in order to buttress our hopes for our own recovery. Healing and everything connected with it has always had a divine aura about it; from the time of Hippocrates and earlier, the healer has occupied a special place in society and been treated with reverence as someone apart from and above the common herd. Even if you tend to a more sceptical view of the medical profession or prefer to say you are realistic – they are human like everyone else – you still want to believe that the experts into whose care you have entrusted yourself really do justify their status and the letters after their name.

The don't-want-to-knows are probably in the minority these days. Certainly most people reading this book are unlikely to be in that category, and this is probably only one of the sources from which you will have been seeking facts and advice to help you make up your mind. The problem today is not so much lack of information – there's plenty of it about if you know how to look for it – but rather how a non-medical person is to absorb a mass of facts and then make the 'right' decision based on a choice between several options.

'When I heard the word cancer I switched off. I thought I had been given a death sentence.'

*Katrina*

This is a very common reaction but it means that when you eventually switch on again, as you obviously will, you may have to go back to your doctor, more than once, to discuss your options. Don't be afraid of wasting his or her time - ask for an appointment if you need it. It's a good idea to make a list beforehand of the questions you want to ask. Ask your partner or a good friend to accompany you who can put questions on your behalf, if you like, and, just as important, hear the things the doctor tells you which may still elude you. You may, however, prefer to talk to the doctor on your own, or you may have no choice but to do so.

'Before he started, he asked me why I had come alone. "Most people bring someone to hold their hand," he said. I had no idea he was going to tell me I had cancer. Then he told me I could have either a mastectomy or a lumpectomy but that he strongly advised me to have a mastectomy. He wanted me to make up my mind on the spot and was annoyed when I insisted I had to have time to think it over. I was divorced and alone and it was two days before Christmas. I left thinking I'd be dead in a month.'

*Fern*

Obviously, if there is a breast care nurse in your hospital, she is the ideal person to whom you can talk about whatever's worrying you. You can use her as a sounding board to test out your thoughts without feeling you are taking up a busy person's time. Her time is your time and she is there just to help you. But if there isn't such a person in your hospital, you may have to look among friends or family for someone who is willing to let you talk through your problems, and discuss the options that have been presented to you.

There was a recent interesting experiment conducted by a psychologist and a surgeon to see whether tape-recording the surgeon's talk to the patient would help. The interview started with the surgeon breaking the bad news; he then continued by describing further tests and the various surgical options; and it ended with him providing the patient with relevant information about radiotherapy and chemotherapy. Everything was in the interview that a patient might expect to hear on her first visit, yet very little of which she is likely to retain, given her state of mind.

The patients in this study were then given the tape so that they could, in the privacy of their own homes, re-run it as often as they liked. It proved to have many benefits, of both a psychological and practical nature.

The psychological aspects first: it spared the patient the pain and distress of having to repeat to other people several times over what the doctor had told her. It also helped many of the women to calm down, collect their thoughts and start to feel more positive about their future as they really heard for the first time what the doctor was telling them. Everyone who was asked to listen to it could also hear for themselves exactly what had been said, enabling them to understand the situation much more directly. This must surely have helped many of them to offer more appropriate support.

From a practical angle its supreme benefit lay in enabling the patient to remember points she might have forgotten, and to clarify those she had heard but not really comprehended the first time round. There were advantages for the surgeon too. It must have cut down considerably on the time he would otherwise have had to give to patients and possibly their relatives as well, requesting further explanations. If necessary, he could simply refer them to the tape, having run through it on his own before talking to the patient in order to remind himself of what he had said.

It's to be hoped that more doctors will try this out. It won't work well for everyone, whether they be patient or doctor, if only because some people feel uneasy handling a tape recorder or knowing that what they say is being recorded, but for those who are not put off by a bit of technology, it could be worth a try. For doctors, there is the further advantage in that it enables them to check up on their own style of delivery. Listening to one's recorded voice is always a salutary experience, and never more so than when conducting an interview.

If you are a particularly self-confident sort of person and feel you have a sufficiently good relationship with your doctor to dare to ask, you might like to suggest that you bring a tape recorder to your next meeting instead of a notebook. Be prepared, though, for some less than sympathetic reactions. Even the apparently mature and friendly doctor may feel you are putting him or her on the spot and respond defensively. 'Don't you trust me?' is the reaction one woman got when she began asking some quite simple questions; to a doctor who is as paranoid as that, the mere sight of a tape recorder could seriously jeopardize an already fragile patient–doctor relationship.

This is not the time for patients to be challenging their doctors or feeling challenged themselves. Unfortunately, because communication skills are low down on the priority list at medical school, many doctors emerge from their training quite unaware how deficient they are in this respect. Being a good communicator does, of course, have quite a lot to do with personality and some people, almost without trying, are going to do it much better than others. Experience is also a great teacher but, unfortunately, you may be one of the patients on whom the doctor is doing the learning. If you are having serious problems in this respect, don't suffer in silence. You may not be able to get any further with your own doctor, but you can get help from organizations which offer a telephone helpline and can even introduce you to a counsellor if that seems appropriate (see chapter ten).

## Giving Informed Consent

In normal circumstances, you think of yourself as an autonomous being, responsible for your actions and relatively free to make your own decisions on matters affecting your life and your wellbeing. Obviously, it is never quite as simple and straightforward as we would like to believe, because none of us is an island. We live in a society; our way of life depends to a great extent on our abiding by the common consent that we will try to keep within the boundaries and obey the laws, if only to make life tolerable for us as much as for everyone else. We also live within a smaller, much more relevant microcosm - the overlapping worlds of work, family, friends and acquaintances - and here again our choices and decisions will often be affected by other people; the closer they are, the greater their influence is likely to be.

To be diagnosed with a life-threatening disease puts you, as we have already said, into another world - the unfamiliar arena of hospitals, doctors, and a multitude of other health professionals, many of them operating high-tech machinery and speaking an incomprehensible jargon. You are at the centre of all this, the focus of their attention and yet you can easily feel that you are becoming dehumanized and alienated; other people are turning you into an object rather than a person.

'I felt like something thrown off the end of a conveyor belt. At no time did anyone sit down and talk to me about cancer or any other problems.'

*Isobel*

Even if there are people around who invite you to talk to them, like the breast care nurse, not every patient wants to take advantage of that offer in a hospital setting. Whatever your personal inclination, the mere fact of being a patient immediately puts you at a considerable disadvantage. However much you struggle to understand what is going on around you and why certain things are being done to you, you still feel ignorant and confused. You have been told that you are seriously ill, even though you may not feel it, and you are devastated by that knowledge. This fact alone makes you feel extremely vulnerable, and immediately puts you in a weak position from which to engage in a relationship with your doctor, one where you would feel at least as competent to discuss your options for action as you would, say, with a lawyer or a bank manager. All three are professionals, experts in their field, which is why you consult them, but the patient is dependent on the doctor in a far more crucial life-or-death way than clients are with either of the other two.

At the beginning of this chapter we talked about the feeling of losing control that so many people experience after a diagnosis of cancer. Information gathering is one way to overcome that sense of helplessness, but once you've got all the information, what are you going to do with it? How can you use it?

In the orthodox health care situation it is largely a matter of first trying to understand what is being offered to you; then making the basic decision whether you're going to ask your doctor to select the treatments for you, or whether you are going to insist on being involved, step by step, throughout the decision-making process. If you choose the latter option, you have declared your determination to resume the autonomy you felt you had lost when you entered the hospital, but it may not always be an easy path to follow. For one thing, you will always remain dependent on the willingness and the reliability of those looking after you to respect your wishes to be kept informed at all times.

As we know, doctors vary considerably in their ability to communicate. Some doctors are pleased to explain what's going on because they see it as a way of helping the patient towards recovery. This holistic attitude would seem to make sense and is borne out by research. A patient who understands why certain treatments are being suggested and what to expect from them - the side effects as well as the benefits - usually feels more encouraged to stick with the regimen even when at times it can be quite unpleasant. Doctors who are more reluctant about imparting information may take a mechanistic view of medicine; they really aren't too bothered how the patient feels so long as she accepts the treatment. Others, however, are deliberately 'economical with the truth' because they genuinely think it's kinder. They are the paternalists (not always male) who believe that it can be seriously harmful for the patient to know too much about their illness or to involve them in making decisions which they might later regret.

'In the end I left it to the doctor to decide the treatment, but I was glad I had been asked if I wanted to choose.'
*Julia*

It's up to you, the patient, to decide how much you want to know and how deeply you wish to be involved. Even if you feel that on the whole you would prefer the doctor to take the responsibility for your treatment, never allow yourself to be persuaded to sign anything unless you are sure you know why you are doing it, and that you understand to what you are consenting. If the consent form presented to you before your operation, or any other treatment you may have, contains a phrase suggesting that you agree you have been 'fully informed', look your doctor in the eye and ask whether that is true.

Too many people, the British in particular, are meek and passive patients, anxious to please and not to cause a fuss, traits which have allowed doctors far too much freedom to decide on our behalf what's best for us. Always remember that it's your body you are signing over. You can think of the consent form as a kind of receipt from the doctor, confirming that during this period of temporary surrender for 'repair' only what has been agreed between you will be done. Don't, under any circumstances, consent to vague wording which allows the doctor to do further surgery 'should it be considered necessary' unless, of course, that's what you really want. For the same reasons, never agree to take part in a research study unless you are sure you know what it's about and why you have been asked. If you don't want medical students or other observers present at your operation, you can strike out that clause.

Sometimes the consent form is produced at a very late stage and it may be a junior doctor who has been deputed to ask you to sign it. Whoever it is, if the doctor can't answer your questions satisfactorily, you have a right to ask for another doctor to come and explain the precise terms of your consent to you. If you are still not happy, then the form will have to be re-worded in a version that suits what you are prepared to sign. This sounds more difficult than it is in practice. If you explain your reasons quietly but firmly, the doctors will have to listen. No-one can force you to sign something you don't want to and, from every point of view, it's much easier to deal with patients who are satisfied that they are fully in the picture.

## What Else Can I Do For Me?

Up to now we have discussed only the orthodox treatments that will be offered to you by hospital consultants. There are a few people who, after hearing what is available in orthodox medicine, may decide they want nothing of it and look elsewhere for treatment. They may settle for one particular alternative treatment or, more typically, they may pick and choose among various therapies. Obviously what everyone hopes for is a cure, but no one can guarantee such an outcome from whatever part of the healing spectrum they come - orthodox, alternative or somewhere in the middle.

There have always been charlatans, quacks and confidence tricksters in every branch of medicine who have taken advantage of people's fears for their own (usually mercenary) ends. Whatever their motives, and sometimes they are dangerously misguided rather than corrupt, it's sensible to be cautious of anyone who claims certainty in such an unpredictable area. The doctor who says 'we got it all out in time' is not being really honest with the patient because no-one can ever be completely sure; it's much wiser to say something like 'we hope . . .' To offer a false assurance which can't be guaranteed is behaving not much better than the alternative practitioner who promises a cure to the client providing he or she obediently, and often at some considerable personal cost, follows whatever the special diet or nostrum may be.

On the other hand, it has been known for remission or even cure to occur in cases where the doctors may have tried everything and given up all hope, irrespective of whether the patient had been receiving complementary treatment as well. Another even more familiar situation is that of two patients, apparently presenting with the same type and stage of cancer and receiving the same treatment, yet one thrives and the other goes downhill rapidly. All in the mind? That's not as offbeat as it sounds.

Positive thinking has been shown to enhance the long-term survival of cancer patients in more than one controlled psychological study. It makes sense, after all. If you are determined to beat your disease you are summoning up all your defences, your immune system in other words, to make a counterattack. Although we still understand so little about how the mind-body interaction works, we have plenty of empirical evidence to show that the mind, especially when focused in a trained way, can and does control the body to a remarkable extent. Meditation, visualization, dream therapy and relaxation are all ways of working with your mind to restore and heal your body.

These methods produce several benefits. First of all, they have a direct physical impact by calming and releasing the tensions and general sense of dis-ease (quite different from feeling ill) which have been invading you and making it difficult for you to think straight. They also sustain you and strengthen you psychologically by helping you to recover some control over your own life. Although you may still have to accept in a passive way the medical treatments that you have been told offer you the best chance of getting better, there is now something extra you can do for yourself. Last but not least, and it's probably the most usual reason for many people, the complementary treatments, generally speaking, have one great advantage over orthodox treatments: they actually make you feel better. That is important, particularly if you face the prospect of an exhausting regimen like chemotherapy or radiotherapy. In chapter seven various complementary therapies especially suitable for cancer patients are described.

At this stage, probably your best course is to continue with anything you may already be doing, relaxation, for instance, or yoga. If there's something you have always wanted to try, now could be the moment. The effort expended and the concentration in learning something new will help you to forget for a while your other problems, and you may be surprised how soon you find it also helps you to cope better with them. It is also a good preparation for going into hospital and having surgery. An operation is always a stressful event, so it's important to build up your physical and mental reserves beforehand.

# 5

## LOSS AND RECOVERY

### Mourning

'Before I went into hospital I said goodbye to myself. I stood in front of the mirror and looked at myself. To remember. After surgery, when the bandage had come off, I went into the bathroom, looked at myself and wept.'

*Jinty*

Only the woman who has been through this experience can know what it feels like and say it as it is. Those moving words were spoken to me by Jinty Blanckenhagen in an interview which appeared on 7th October 1986 in the first issue of the *Independent* newspaper. By then it was many years after her mastectomy and she was leading an exceptionally full life, doing the balancing act between home and work that so many women are familiar with: in her case it involved looking after home, husband and three teenage daughters on the one hand, and being full-time director of the Breast Care and Mastectomy Association on the other.

Her need to acknowledge her loss and give herself time to grieve was something that Jinty had to discover for herself. She had accepted the prospect of a mastectomy with a heavy heart but unreservedly, shutting out any lingering hopes that the operation could be more conservative. The doctor had convinced her there was no alternative, and she had far too much to live for to want to waste any energy in futile regrets. For Jinty, as for most women caught in this situation, her survival was uppermost in her mind. That said, no one should minimize the trauma of losing a breast.

A woman's bosom is an integral part of her sense of herself. She will have been aware of it ever since her breasts first began budding. She has probably watched them develop with a host of conflicting feelings - apprehension, delight, eagerness, dissatisfaction - and more. Her breasts contribute to her identity in so many ways - as lover, mother, friend - woman of any age, married or single, walking down the street or into a crowded room, buying clothes, hugging a child, feeding a baby, embracing a lover. Her breasts are her: not all of her but enough to make her feel that she is losing something that really matters when a breast is amputated. The breasts are not limbs, and they don't have the same obvious functional importance, but they have another significance which goes far deeper than merely their appearance.

'Old friends, that's what they were,' one unmarried woman, who had two mastectomies over a period of three years, confided to me. 'They had been with me everywhere; they were part of me. I loved them and my lovers loved them. To lose one was bad enough. When the second went it was terrible. Of course, I got over it. You do, but it took a long time.' She subsequently had a reconstruction which, though not perfect from the cosmetic point of view, made her feel happier about herself.

Whether the removal is partial or total is not always the greatest concern; however much or little it is, what matters more is that something quite personal and special is to be taken away from you, never to be returned. You must be allowed to mourn that loss. It is a genuine bereavement, and needs to be recognized as such and respected. For some women there is also a sense of outrage; it can feel almost as if you have been assaulted, and these feelings may be intensified if a woman has additional worries about her partner's reaction. Some men can be very possessive about their partner's body. The breasts particularly seem to inspire a kind of fierce macho pride which in the good times a woman may have exulted in, but in the bad times, like now, may terrify her.

Will he reject me? Will he stop loving me? Will I ever find anyone to love me again? What will my children think of me? Will I look a freak? Questions and fears like these go through the minds of most women confronting the prospect of breast surgery. Women on their own are not immune from them either. Young or old, and whatever she may say for public consumption, it is a rare woman who does not care deeply about her breasts.

Fortunately, these fears of rejection are often groundless and many women find, to their amazement and joy, that it turns out quite the reverse: their marriage or relationship is actually deepened and enhanced by this crisis. Or they may make a new and better relationship with someone who never knew them with two breasts. The shadow of loss which hovers over two people may also bring them closer together, although before that happens there may be a temporary period of estrangement while the partner goes through his or her own dark night of the soul. It's often forgotten that cancer is a crisis which affects everyone who comes into contact with it. Sometimes the relatives and close friends need almost as much support and counselling as the patient; sometimes they may even need more.

None of this help was available in the late 1970s when Jinty had her mastectomy, nor indeed was it to be for some years afterwards. Women just had to cope somehow, and most hid away their grief and depression as best they could, because

cancer was something you did not talk about. Even today, with
so much more help available, it is estimated that about a
quarter of the women who have surgery for breast cancer
become clinically depressed, and many more remain in a low
state for a long time. Much of this unhappiness could be
avoided if they were able to find professional help to support
them through their time of loss. (See chapter ten for more
information about such resources.)

Jinty was fortunate to have a devoted husband who assured
her right from the start that he would always be there, and
that it made absolutely no difference to him whether she had
two breasts, one or none. She would always be the woman
he had loved and married and would go on loving. Even so,
with hindsight, she would have liked to have been able to talk
to someone like a breast care nurse who could explain the
medical details to her. The surgeon, though esteemed for his
technical skills, lacked warmth and sympathy.

'He didn't talk much himself and he made it clear that he
thought I was doubting him if I asked questions'. Unnerved
by his detachment, she wondered rather desperately where
she could turn. There was so much more she did need to
know. For instance, none of the doctors had warned her that
the oopherectomy (removal of the ovaries) which they advised
her to have shortly after the mastectomy would bring on
menopausal symptoms. It had been bad enough just to be told
rather casually by the senior registrar that it was thought to
be a necessary operation.

'I let the side down and howled. The sister was very cross
with me and told me to pull myself together because the
consultant was coming. They couldn't understand why I
should mind so much when I'd already got three children, but
I'd wanted one more. In the end I signed the form because
it was put to me that it was a very good treatment.'

So indeed it has proved to be - for Jinty who had 11 years

of remission - and many others as we now know from the results of the recent overview described in chapter three. But how many women of her age - she was still in her thirties - have been through the same needless shock and distress as they begin to suffer hot flushes and night sweats and find themselves feeling anxious about coping? 'I felt old - my skin was dry and my hair lank - and it made me very depressed for a while.' She believed she could have been spared some of these extra worries if there had just been someone to talk to who would have been able to give her practical advice and information.

'Your friends try very hard and you know they want to help you but there are things you really can't say to them. They wouldn't understand and you don't want to upset them.'
*Judy*

Eventually Jinty did find a confidante, a kind voice at the end of a telephone line who told her she did understand how she was feeling because she had been through a similar experience herself, but she could assure her that in the end it would be all right. And here she was to prove it, all these years later, looking good and feeling well. The voice belonged to Betty Westgate, founder of the Mastectomy Association (the original name of the organization), who until then had been running it virtually single-handed. Jinty never forgot the relief and happiness - yes, that is the right word to use - that she felt after putting down the telephone. There was a woman out there who didn't think she was being either silly or weak. She had been through the same thing herself and she understood what Jinty was feeling. She even had answers to the practical questions no-one in hospital had seemed able to answer, like where you could find a decent prosthesis. (More about that in chapter eight.)

# Before The Operation

The tests will all have been done and the operation date is fixed. Now you just have to make sure that everything is organized for the days that you are to spend in hospital.

You will have had to ask your employer for time off, but whether you explain why is, obviously, up to you. Most employers these days are sufficiently enlightened to know that an operation for cancer, though of course serious, doesn't mean that you won't be able to work again. Some employers can be very positive and supportive and will give you all the help they can and plenty of time to recuperate. Others may be rather grudging by comparison and you may feel under some pressure to return to work as quickly as possible. And there will always be a few who seem still to be back in the Dark Ages, and who behave as if cancer were a deadly and contagious disease. It would be nice in an ideal world if you could show them by your frank attitude that this is not the case but clearly, you don't want to jeopardize your job. What you decide to do in such circumstances is entirely up to you, and no-one should influence you to say anything you would prefer to leave unsaid.

If you have a family you will have made the usual domestic arrangements and found someone to look after your children, preferably a grandparent or other relative if their father is not around or feels he can't manage on his own. To some extent it depends on the age of your children how much you decide to tell them, but it's probably wiser to tell them more rather than less. Children are very sensitive at picking up atmospheres, and if they suspect you are hiding something from them it may cause them to feel frightened and even guilty. A young child may imagine that Mummy is going into hospital because it has been naughty; an older one may have the same kind of fear, but be too ashamed to admit it and cover up by being rude or aggressive.

'I don't know whether I handled it right. I told them about good cells and bad cells and talked to them a lot about everything. They were still very small [four and two] but the older one was very interested. I do wonder though whether I overburdened them. Do they go round thinking their mother could drop dead? I just know that's the way I had to do it.'

*Vera*

The best you can do for your children is to reassure them that when you come home you will be the same Mum you were before you went into hospital. You may not always feel quite like that, but here a little bit of the-show-must-go-on spirit is in order. Children need to feel that they are secure. If it's not possible for them to visit you in hospital, try and keep in contact by sending cards or calling them on the telephone.

Isobel, who also had two young daughters when she was first diagnosed and, like Vera, didn't believe in hiding anything from them, still chuckles today when she remembers the card her older daughter sent her. 'It said "sorry for your loss" which expressed what she felt for me but when I opened it up, it was a card meant for someone who's had a death in the family.' Isobel was only 32 when she had her first mastectomy and she didn't think she'd live to see her daughters grow up. Fifteen years later, she's enjoying spoiling her first grandson.

If you are living on your own there may be all sorts of practical arrangements to make, like stopping the milk and newspapers, leaving a spare set of keys with a neighbour, asking a friend to water your plants or feed the cat. These are all finicky details, the sort of things you have to do before going on holiday, but they take up time and they can be bothersome.

'I was glad I was on my own. I think I would have found it very difficult to take the strain of someone else's worry as well as my own. I told just one friend beforehand but afterwards I told my sister, and then it was lovely to stay with her and her family and be spoilt and fussed over.'

*Jean*

Make lists if it helps you; one, for instance, for your hospital bag. You will need all the things you would want for an overnight stay anywhere, although in this case it's going to be several days: nightwear, dressing gown and slippers, sponge bag, make-up and so on. Don't forget to put in the things that you know will make you feel good, or comforted, like family photographs, a favourite scent, magazines or a novel you've been longing to read. Choose at least one pretty nightdress and bring in a bra which fits you well, but it should not be too tight, or underwired. The hospital may send you a patient leaflet which briefly outlines what to expect and any requirements they may have.

Once arrived and undressed, you will have various routine checks for blood pressure, heart and lungs. A medical history will be taken to make sure that nothing unusual has been overlooked and that the medication is not going to upset any other condition you may have. Both the surgeon and the anaesthetist may visit you to discuss the operation. This is your opportunity to ask all the last-minute questions you want. Don't be timid! You have enough to think about without having some nagging worry at the back of your mind to which there is probably quite a simple answer. At some stage you will also be asked to sign the consent form which was discussed in chapter four. Again, ask all you want and don't allow yourself to be rushed into signing until everything has been explained to your satisfaction.

This is an anxious time for you. You may ordinarily be rather good at putting yourself into a state of relaxation, but it could be more difficult on this occasion. If this is the case it might be sensible to take the sleeping tablets that the nurse will offer you. A good night's sleep is also a good preparation for recovery.

## After The Operation

When you wake up after your operation you will find you have some kind of dressing over the incision. It could be a light bandage or a sticking plaster. It really depends on the operation you have had. You may feel a bit wired up like a puppet on a string with tubes apparently protruding all over the place, but it's not as bad as it may seem. The drip in your hand or arm is replacing fluid lost during surgery so that you don't become dehydrated. The tubes coming from the incision on your chest, and also from under your arm if you have had lymph nodes removed, are there to drain any surplus fluid and so hasten the healing process. These tubes have to stay in place for a few days which means walking around with them, because you will be encouraged to get up and start moving as soon as possible. One way of coping is to put the drainage bottles containing the tubes into plastic carrier bags which you can hold, and when you need to go to the toilet a nurse will push the drip stand behind you. You will be able to have a bath quite quickly, providing you keep the dressing dry.

Some people get very nauseated by the anaesthetic and aren't able to eat for a couple of days. If you're really sick you will be given something to quell the nausea. The stitches can cause a feeling of tightness in the chest, and the armpit area where the lymph nodes were removed may also feel somewhat sore and numb. The numbness sometimes lasts for a few months, but this is nothing to worry about. People's pain thresholds vary, but if you're in any discomfort this is no time to be a martyr. It's easy to ask for a painkiller and, as your morale lifts, so will your road to recovery speed up.

The length of time you need to spend in hospital usually depends on the extent of your operation. If it's a lumpectomy it may only be for a couple of days, but if you have had reconstruction following a mastectomy or are starting a course of chemotherapy immediately, then it could be twelve days to a fortnight. Providing there are no complications like infection, the tubes will come out within a week and the stitches after eight to 10 days. Neither of these procedures is painful. The skin may thicken slightly as it heals but again, this is perfectly normal.

## Ups And Downs

As you can see, in most people the physical effects are relatively mild but there may be more dramatic emotional and psychological reactions.

> 'I was so relieved just to be alive. I felt quite euphoric. Then I came down with a crash.'
>
> *Katrina*

It's quite usual for a woman to have mood swings veering from elation to depression at a time like this. You feel wonderful because the operation you dreaded so much is behind you. Everything else will surely be easy from now on. Katrina had been convinced that she would never survive the anaesthetic. Not that she had any good reason to think this; ironically, it was probably just because she was a such a healthy woman, in her mid-thirties, who had never been ill before, but she associated hospital with her mother's death.

'The surgeon was marvellous. He saw me before I went in

and held my hand, and he was there the minute I came round. I felt so pleased to have survived it. I thought the worst part was over and that now I could face up to any other treatment.' Despite all the support from hospital staff, which she acknowledges to have been outstanding – the nurses would come and sit with her and talk to her even during the night – she still couldn't avoid moments of feeling overwhelmed by depression and fear.

Vera and Katrina both had mothers who died relatively young of breast cancer, and this naturally makes them feel particularly threatened. But their hospital experiences were very different. Whereas Katrina felt she was surrounded by people who understood her fears, Vera found that the support she was given, though well-meaning, often jarred because it seemed to make light of her anxieties.

'I was on a surgical ward where there were four of us with cancer. We never talked to each other about what we felt. One woman said to me that she was going to tell everyone she had her appendix out. I felt very angry that this was happening to me, and basically I was terrified. I thought I was dying and I didn't want all these chirpy people round me, telling me to buck up. I cried a lot and made a lot of fuss and I expect they thought I was pathetic, but I thought they ought to have been more understanding. There was just one nurse who did try and we talked about my mother. I appreciated that.'

It's important to feel you can express your emotions openly: crying, getting angry, admitting fear, mourning your mutilation, are all absolutely normal reactions in the circumstances. It would be strange if you didn't have these feelings, and you shouldn't feel embarrassed about showing them. That may be easier said than done, of course, as Vera discovered, or it may go against your particular grain if you have always been a reserved person. In Vera's case, it was only after she left hospital that she was able to find the support she needed by joining a self-help group and getting some counselling through BACUP.

## How Will I Look?

Looking at your scar for the first time is probably the most difficult thing you will have to do after your operation. Many women ask a nurse to be present to help them. Another way of doing it is to stand in front of the mirror (like Jinty) and look at it that way. The impact is less direct than looking down.

> 'I thought I'd prepared myself beforehand but it was still a shock to see the breast had gone. Once the discolouration went, it wasn't so bad. My husband was marvellous. He just undid the bandage and kissed the scar.'
>
> *Margaret*

It can be better than you had hoped. Katrina, who had a lumpectomy, recalls: 'I was amazed to see how neat it was. There were no visible stitches. I felt so relieved.'

Most doctors now try very hard to make the scar as tidy and unobtrusive as possible. If you have a mastectomy, your chest will be flat on the side where the breast and nipple have been removed. The scar will be either horizontal or diagonal depending on the position of the tumour. Your chest is unlikely to look hollowed unless, for some reason, like having a large tumour fixed to the chest wall, a lot of underlying chest muscle had to be removed. The aim of a lumpectomy is to reduce the disfigurement, so the scar should be fairly small. If you are lucky, and the tumour is situated in a position where the surgeon is able to cut round underneath the lower curve of your breast, it may be almost invisible. This is the kind of cut a doctor planning a subcutaneous reconstruction (see chapter six) will also try to do.

In hospital you should be offered a temporary breast form to wear attached inside your bra. You don't have to wear it, but it's very light and suitable for women who have had either a mastectomy or some kinds of lumpectomy. As well as restoring your shape, it also protects your scar while it is still tender. You can wear this breast form at night as well. Later, when the scar is completely healed, you will be able to wear a heavier, more realistic breast form, made of silicone, and called a prosthesis. In the UK these are available through the National Health Service as well as from commercial stockists. If there is no breast care nurse in your hospital, someone called an appliance officer will visit you while you are still in the ward to measure you and make an appointment for a fitting at a later date as an out-patient.

Another hospital visitor is the physiotherapist, who will teach you some exercises to help you recover the full use of your arm on the operated side. It's very important to continue doing these when you go home so that you can quickly regain your full flexibility. (Prostheses and exercises are described in greater detail in chapter eight).

## Coming Home

'When I came back home I needed to think that I could do things for myself, even little things like shopping. I didn't want to be looked after.'

*Katrina*

You will probably feel some physical after-effects for a few days or even weeks after the operation, but they will wear off eventually. For instance, you may have pins and needles, a light darting sensation across your chest, or a numbness near your scar or under your arm. If there is any redness or a burning sensation in the scar region, report it to your doctor because this could mean there's an infection. A course of antibiotics will soon clear it up.

The shoulder on the side of the operated breast may feel stiff and uncomfortable, particularly if you have had a mastectomy or your lymph glands removed. Routine actions like brushing and combing your hair will help to loosen it up, but some things like driving the car or doing a sport like tennis or golf may be more difficult. Take things slowly, a bit at a time. You don't have to prove anything to anyone.

As a general rule, try to use your arm as normally as possible after surgery, but do avoid heavy housework or lifting for at least the first six weeks. Keep doing the exercises which you learnt in hospital (see chapter eight).

After a mastectomy it may help to sleep with your arm on a pillow for a few weeks. Should your arm become swollen, don't delay telling your doctor, because this will certainly require treatment. There are ways you can look after your arm and hand to prevent it developing into a chronic condition called lymphoedema. (See chapter nine.)

'After the initial high of feeling that I was in good hands
– I was getting the very best of care in a well-known hospital
– I had a depression on returning home.'

*Sue*

This is a very common reaction. In the hospital you will have been cocooned by attentive medical staff and visits from your family and friends. You won't have been expected to think about anything other than making a good recovery. But when you return home, even though it is to familiar surroundings, there will also be the routine tasks to do and problems to face that you had temporarily forgotten.

Whether you live alone, with a partner or have a busy family life, there are going to be times when you feel isolated and low. You may be finding it harder to cope because you get exhausted very easily. This will almost certainly be true if you are having further treatment like radiotherapy or chemotherapy.

Pamper yourself. Take things gently at first and be sensible about how much you do. Rest periods are helpful in these early days, but it's also a good thing to start picking up the threads again - seeing friends, perhaps taking a holiday before returning to work. Everything you do should be at the pace which suits you, not to fit in with anyone else's demands.

Gradually, as your physical strength returns, you should begin to feel as fit as you were before the operation, physically at any rate. Sometimes, though, you will feel fatigue and a lassitude which has more to do with your state of mind than your body. It's hardly surprising that you should feel depressed after all you have been through.

'Every time I looked down at myself I was reminded of what had happened to me and I cried.'

*Margaret*

It may be that you decide the time has come to make some major changes in your life, for instance, finding a new job or even making a complete career change. Many people do, and are grateful to the cancer for having pushed them into it. Or it may be you have a rocky relationship that no longer seems worth fighting for. Whatever the change may be, don't rush at it. Time becomes very precious after a brush with mortality, and you don't want to waste a moment of it, but this period at home - on your own perhaps for quite a lot of the day - offers you a breathing space between hospital and the hustling world outside which soon enough will suck you back.

Meanwhile, taking the time to reflect and ponder, enjoy small pleasures and see things with new eyes is all part of your recovery. You have a chance to take stock of your life and make quiet plans for the future. Don't miss it.

Your friends and family will be very important to you, but however supportive they want to be, there are going to be times when you feel they don't really understand what you are going through. Perhaps you think they are being over-protective, or so anxious on your behalf that it makes it very difficult to have a normal conversation. Alternatively, perhaps they imagine that now you are home and the operation is behind you, life can go back to what it was before you were ill. But you may not find it so easy. Life is not the same, and you are not the person you were.

It's hard for them because they love you and your illness has frightened them. But it's also hard for you because you may feel you have to be strong for them as well as yourself, or pretend to be what you no longer are. This effort can become an intolerable burden and if it does, then it's important you seek some outside help. The solution may lie in something as simple as joining a support group or talking on the telephone to a BCMA volunteer, or you may need some professional cancer counselling. (See chapter ten.)

# 6

## WHAT ABOUT BREAST RECONSTRUCTION?

### Is Breast Reconstruction Safe?

This has to be the first question you ask yourself today, given the unfavourable publicity that breast implants have recently received. It's not an easy one to answer because all the information is still not to hand, so the best anyone can do at the moment is to consider the evidence there is, consult widely and then make up their own mind. The final responsibility has to be yours.

It was only at the beginning of the eighties that breast reconstruction after a mastectomy became widely available on the NHS. This coincided with a dawning realization among the more perceptive doctors that many of their cancer patients were finding it exceedingly hard to recover from the psychological effects of a mastectomy. Their sense of loss was undoubtedly not helped by the widespread lack of support at the time. Many women were plunged into despair because they felt that an essential part of their womanhood had been destroyed, and those doctors who realized this believed that by offering a breast reconstruction, they could also offer new hope.

Hitherto, most surgeons had tended to regard breast reconstruction as a frivolity, something only a vain woman would request. You had to be exceptionally brave and determined to ask for it, unless your doctor happened to be one of the few known to be in favour of it. Today it is unusual for a doctor to refuse it to a patient, and if he or she does so without giving a good medical reason, you can always ask for a second opinion.

A breast reconstruction usually, but not always, involves having a silicone implant. This is a transparent, malleable bag containing silicone gel which mimics the softness and mobility of a woman's breast. The same implant is used for women having their breast size increased for cosmetic reasons. Breast augmentation is, of course, an operation that plastic surgeons have been doing for a long time, and it forms a large portion of their private practice. Breast reconstruction, for reasons which will become clear later in this chapter, is usually a more complicated procedure, so when general surgeons first became interested in what their colleagues were doing for healthy women, they realized that they would have to develop new techniques. Some have now made it a speciality they can offer as part of a total package to women facing surgery for breast cancer; others will do the mastectomy but leave the reconstruction to a plastic surgeon.

Today, there are 100,000 British women who have had breast implants, 60,000 of whom have had breast reconstructions. Most of these women are pleased with their replacement breasts, even if they aren't always perfect replicas of the original. At the end of 1991 they and their doctors were thrown into a state of ferment because the American Food and Drugs Administration (FDA) issued a ruling which imposed a 45 day voluntary moratorium on the supplying or use of these implants while new data was evaluated. Behind the terse officialese lay a story of mounting confusion spiked with hysteria as American women reported stories of exploding or leaking implants. It was being suggested that in some cases the implants had caused cancer in other organs, and that they might also be responsible for breaking down the auto-immune system.

The British doctors, led by the Chief Medical Officer, Dr Kenneth Calman, decided to hold their fire until more evidence was produced. Up to the time of writing, neither they nor many of their European colleagues have been sufficiently convinced by what has emerged across the Atlantic to suggest either stopping implant surgery or removing those implants already in place. They have repeatedly said that there is no evidence for the kind of horrific situations depicted on television programmes such as the UK's *World in Action* (23rd September 1991 and February 1992). All the same, they continue to keep an open mind on the subject, and further evidence from the United States, whether good or bad, will undoubtedly have a crucial bearing on future decisions elsewhere. At the end of February 1992 the FDA renounced its ban on the use of silicone breast implants, having studied the research in depth and concluded there was insufficient evidence to support the claim that they posed a health risk.

Although it has apparently always been known that silicone tends to leak small amounts into other parts of the body, British doctors have taken the view that this is so minimal it can cause no damage. There is no evidence to show that cancer is caused by this leakage, either as a new primary in the breast or one appearing in other parts of the body. Another fear has been that the presence of an implant would mask the growth of a new tumour if it was sited behind the implant. Again this fear seems to be unfounded and it is apparently quite possible to do an effective mammogram for screening purposes of a breast containing an implant. You should, however, always make sure the radiographer knows you have one. In the past there has been some doubt about the possible cancer-inducing effect of those silicone implants which are covered with a polyurethane coating. This substance was introduced as a way of counteracting the tendency of implants to become rigid (see below). However, this material has a tendency to break down in the body, and in rats it produces a carcinogenic chemical called TDA. Although this effect has not been found in human beings, and this was confirmed by the Committee on Carcinogenicity in the UK in 1991, the manufacturers decided to withdraw it.

As far as auto-immune disease is concerned, the jury is still out on this one. There has recently been a notorious case in America where the plaintiff cited her breast implants as cause of her crippling arthritis, but here there is a clash of medical opinion because some doctors are saying her disease was present before the implants were inserted. So far, there are no indications that anyone is bringing a similar case in the UK.

A point that tends to be left out of these debates is that the quality of silicone implant varies quite considerably. A leading plastic surgeon in this country warns that they can be anything from top grade specification to something 'quite nasty - leaky and oily' that might have been produced in someone's garage or in the laboratory behind an entrepreneurial chemist's shop. Although it's unlikely to be of such poor quality in an NHS breast reconstruction operation, he would advise any woman contemplating a breast reconstruction which involves a silicone implant to ask her surgeon what make it is. Indeed, she should insist on inspecting it for herself so that she can be satisfied about its shape and its feel, in much the same way that she would want to feel happy about an external prosthesis. This is, after all, a foreign object which is to be lodged in her body indefinitely, for the purpose of simulating her lost breast.

She should certainly not have the experience of this woman

who was told by her surgeon that he would do a mastectomy first and follow it up in a few months time with an implant.

'I woke up and found that I had an implant already put in. When I asked him why he'd changed his mind, he really didn't answer. But doctors don't tell you much, do they?'

*Shirley*

There are some other problems associated with breast implants which, though less sinister, can cause painful and sometimes serious complications. Every woman should be aware of them before she makes up her mind. Certain types of breast reconstruction involve a major displacement of fat and muscle combined with skin grafting; the operation is complex and the healing process can take a long time and be quite uncomfortable. Even where the operation is relatively simple and involves little more than removing breast tissue and inserting a foreign body, this is quite likely to set up a long-term reaction called capsular contracture. This means that fibrous scar tissue forms around the implant, and if it's not counteracted may eventually make the breast become hard and rigid. Should this become too uncomfortable, it may have to be removed and a new implant substituted.

It's one of those strange quirks of medical behaviour that although a good deal of importance is attached, quite rightly, to testing a new drug thoroughly before giving it to patients, the same rigour is not invariably applied to new surgical techniques. There is no record that any studies have been done to compare the different breast reconstruction techniques for such factors as rate and type of complications, cosmetic success, and patient satisfaction. It would have seemed a sensible precaution for doctors at least to be keeping a national register of all their patients with breast reconstructions. This would have enabled them to pick up problems and compare results. Unfortunately, what often happens when things go wrong, in these unmonitored circumstances, is that a woman doesn't go back to the same doctor; instead she seeks out another to rectify the mistakes made by the first one.

## Who Can Have A Breast Reconstruction?

Most women of any age can have this operation either after, or at the same time as surgery for breast cancer, and irrespective of whether it's a total or partial mastectomy, so long as the tumour has not spread too much. If your breasts are large the doctor will probably advise you to have the healthy one reduced somewhat at the same time, because it's not wise for medical reasons to have too heavy a reconstructed breast.

Clearly there are risks as well as benefits attached to breast reconstruction, so it's advisable to consult your doctor very carefully before you make up your mind as to whether or not you want it. Given the present uncertainty about silicone implants, you may decide you want to wait for a bit to see how the situation develops. Some doctors, as a matter of principle, always advise their patients to wait a few months to see how they feel about their missing breast. Often a woman decides she doesn't want to go through yet more operations and adapts well, either to wearing a prosthesis or nothing at all. Radiotherapy is another reason for delaying reconstruction, because the skin needs to recover from the treatment.

Whatever the reasons may be for waiting, if you are at all interested in the idea of having a reconstruction sometime in the future, you should discuss the possibility with your surgeon from the outset. In effect this means well in advance of your mastectomy, because it will influence the way the doctor does your mastectomy. For instance, it's important to try and save the nipple, if at all possible, and to make a scar which will not spoil the final cosmetic result should your breast be reconstructed.

You can feel confident in your doctor if he or she welcomes your caution and is quite happy to show you photographs of previous reconstructions. Many of these women will have had their implants for several years and will be very pleased with the result. Ask also to see pictures of results which the doctor is less pleased about: although the woman depicted may have mixed feelings about the way she looks, she may nonetheless profess herself to be happier to have had the reconstruction rather than have to face life without it. Some women will say they still prefer to have an implant, even though when they're undressed it may look more like a mound than a breast. Under low-cut dresses and swimsuits it gives them a cleavage and looks like the real thing, and that may be their number one priority.

There will, of course, be a small number of women who will be wishing they had never had the operation, although these are not necessarily patients of your doctor. Why not pluck up your courage, and ask him or her about any failures? Most doctors have them and, if they are honest, will own to them. The way your doctor responds to this question could be crucial. A clear explanation and an indication that much has been learnt from the experience could be a greater encouragement to put your faith in your doctor than a whole galaxy of starry successes depicted in photographs that may or may not all be of his work.

## Why Do You Want A Breast Reconstruction?

This is another important question that you must ask: of yourself, obviously, although talking to other people is one of the ways that may help you to find an answer. If you have a partner then surely this must be the first person you consult; it's important to discuss it in depth with each other, as well as together with your doctor. You may also find it helpful to talk it over with a friend or close relative whose opinion you value. The breast care nurse, if there is one in your hospital, is another obvious person because she will be well informed about all types of breast reconstruction and may also be able to introduce you to someone who has had one done which is similar to the one being proposed for you. Alternatively, you could ring the BCMA and ask to be put in touch with a volunteer who has had such a procedure. Whoever it may be, talking to someone who has been through it is the best possible way of learning what it really involves. Here the voice of experience really does count.

But it's not just the physical aspects of breast reconstruction which will concern you. You need to ask yourself why you want to replace the breast you have lost, and what you think this will do for you. This is where a good friend or a wise counsellor can be a wonderful support, because it may be quite painful to explore your own psychological and emotional reasons. It's a situation where you must be prepared to look for the negatives first and then weigh them against the positives. Then you have to ask yourself: are there enough positives to tip the balance in favour of reconstruction despite all the serious negatives?

The known negatives include: the pain and discomfort; the possible long-term ordeal (sometimes it's necessary to have several operations); the side effects and complications, both likely and unlikely; and the possibility of failure or, at best, an unsatisfactory result. The main positive is what you think it will do for you. You may want to have a reconstruction because you think it will save your marriage. That needs thinking about, and maybe you should have some counselling. The most important thing is that whatever you decide, you know that you are doing it for yourself, not for someone else.

It may be that you think reconstruction is essential for your career: you may be a dancer or an actress, or someone like Diana Moran, TV's Green Goddess, who depends on her physique for her career. In her case, with a packed programme stretching months ahead and always on show as a model of health and beauty demonstrating exercise routines, it would have seemed almost unthinkable to have to cope with prostheses. She therefore chose to sign her consent form authorizing the surgeon to do a biopsy to test for cancer which, if positive, was to be followed immediately by bilateral mastectomies and reconstruction, all under the same anaesthetic. She woke up, weeping 'tears of relief and joy to see that it had all been done. I couldn't have faced a second operation immediately afterwards at that time'. Three months later, she was back in full swing, and today probably leads a busier and more demanding life than ever before. She has written her own moving account of her story in her book *A More Difficult Exercise.*

Each woman has her own particular feelings about her breasts. You may think that nothing could ever replace the one you have lost so a reconstruction would be out of the question. Alternatively you may believe that it is just what you need to make you feel better about your appearance, and therefore more reconciled to the fact of cancer. The idea of being able to look down and see a breast where there has always been a breast may be very reassuring, and there are psychological studies to show that women who have a reconstruction immediately after mastectomy seem to recover more rapidly and completely from the emotional trauma. Some would prefer to wait and see how they feel in a few months' time.

'I'm glad my doctor persuaded me to wait a year before having the reconstruction. It gave me time to think about what I was doing, and I got quite used to my prosthesis. I could have lived with it and with only having one breast. I'd tested myself out and I knew I could make new relationships as a single-breasted woman so I didn't lack confidence. I just preferred the idea of not having to fiddle around with a prosthesis in my bra or worrying about losing it when I was swimming.'

Carol

A perfect result can never be guaranteed, so it's important that you do prepare yourself mentally for the possibility that your breast implant may never look quite as good as the breast it replaces. Sometimes it may be difficult to replace the nipple, and you may find it easier to use stick-on nipples. It can be hard for the doctor to match the new breast with the remaining healthy one, and there may be an asymmetry between them which will become even more marked if you either lose or gain a lot of weight. Sometimes the new breast actually looks better than the other one because it is firmer and higher. In such cases the doctor may suggest a small cosmetic operation on the healthy breast: reducing it, perhaps, or lifting the droop slightly.

Most women will find they have few problems following the operation, and the ones they do have will usually clear up quickly. One change which won't go away is that you will have a permanent loss of sensation in your breast, and in your nipple as well if that too has been reconstructed. It's a side effect most women can tolerate with reasonable equanimity, especially if they have been warned to expect it. Sometimes an infection occurs in or around the wound after the operation, but this too can be dealt with quite easily. Calendula cream is particularly recommended to promote healing. All the same, it's best to be prepared for the possibility that the procedure may not turn out to be as straightforward and simple as you had hoped.

# Which Operation?

Your doctor will probably have a preference for a particular operation, usually the one he feels happiest doing and gets the best cosmetic result with, but the final decision will depend on various factors, including the type of mastectomy you have had, any other treatment, and the size and shape of your breasts. It will help your discussion if you are aware of all the options, and the drawbacks and advantages pertaining to each. The procedures have been described here in ascending order of complication, and fall into three main categories.

## 1. SILICONE IMPLANT

This simple procedure, which is similar to the breast augmentation done in healthy women, involves the least trauma and only a short stay in hospital. It is particularly suitable for women who have an early non-invasive cancer (DCIS). Occasionally, it is offered as a preventative measure for women known to be at abnormally high risk of contracting breast cancer.

> 'The saving of a breast, even an imperfect one, also meant the saving of my sanity.'
>
> *Jenny, Observer,* 13th October 1991

### *Method One – Subcutaneous Mastectomy*
The mastectomy and the implant are performed at the same time. The surgeon makes an incision, following the lower curve of the breast, and removes all the tissue, retaining, if possible, the nipple and a layer of fat under the skin. The silicone implant is inserted under the fat and the breast is sewn up. A small silicone implant can also be used to fill out a hollow that may have been left by a lumpectomy or to lift

the opposite healthy breast so that there is a better match between the two.

Sometimes it's not possible to insert the implant at the same time as the mastectomy, because the skin edges may not be very healthy. However, it can probably be done a few days later. The doctor may test the skin with a fluorescent drug which will leave it stained yellow for some time.

One of the advantages of having an implant at the same time as your mastectomy is that you probably won't need any drainage tubes, because the presence of the implant prevents fluid collecting. The drainage tubes are what cause most of the post-operative pain.

The disadvantages of this operation are neither numerous nor serious. If the worst comes to the worst and you eventually develop a tight hard capsule round your implant, it may be necessary to remove it and replace it with another. One experienced surgeon says the problem could be avoided in many more cases, providing the patient is given precise post-operative instructions and follows them carefully. Another problem may occur if the skin is so thin that the implant breaks through. If the surgeon thinks there is a chance this could happen to you, he or she may suggest that you have the following operation instead.

### Method Two – Submuscular Silicone Implant

The same type of implant as described above is placed in a deep pocket on top of the chest wall and under the muscle which covers the chest. The scar follows the line of the mastectomy scar. This implant doesn't give quite as good a result as the 'sub-cut' because the breast mound won't be so pronounced, but it is safe. It is particularly suitable for patients who have had radiotherapy which may affect the quality of the skin and the amount of blood supply flowing to it.

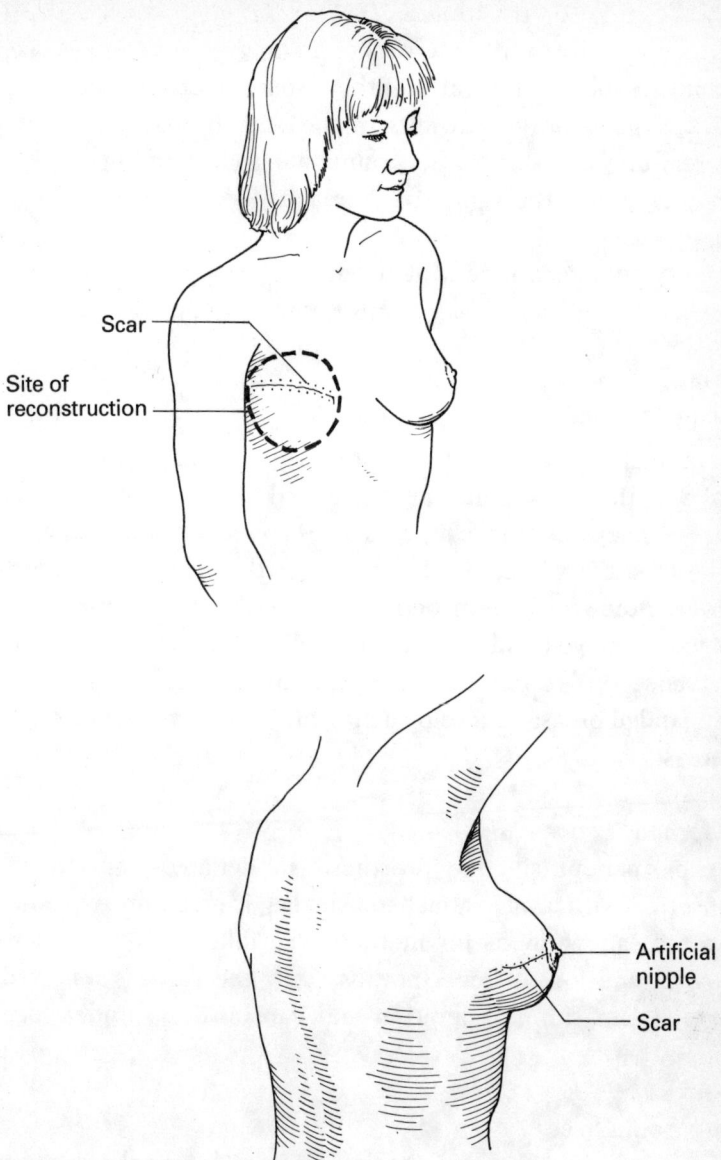

*Fig 5 Submuscular silicone implant.*

## 2. TISSUE EXPANSION

There are three different ways of doing this. Although it takes time - probably several months - some doctors believe that it can give the best results in the end. It works by slowly stretching the skin to accommodate an expanding silicone implant until the right size is reached.

'I would recommend it to anyone.'
*Isobel (who has had both breasts reconstructed by tissue expansion)*

### Method One

An inflatable silicone bag is inserted under the chest muscle. Gradually, on a weekly basis, the bag is expanded by means of a sterile saline solution introduced through a valve under local anaesthetic. This process takes about two months; when the breast has become slightly larger than the other natural breast, the valve is removed. After a further three months the bag is removed and a permanent silicone prosthesis inserted in a second operation. The waiting time allows for the expanded breast to develop a matching droop with the natural breast.

### Method Two

A permanent silicone prosthesis in deflated condition is inserted with a valve attached. The bag is gradually expanded in the same way as for method one, followed by the same waiting period of three months. Only the valve is removed, which is a simple operation and can be done under local anaesthetic.

### Method Three

The implant is changed at regular intervals and the cavity is re-shaped at each change. Although this takes longer and is somewhat troublesome, it enables the surgeon to have more

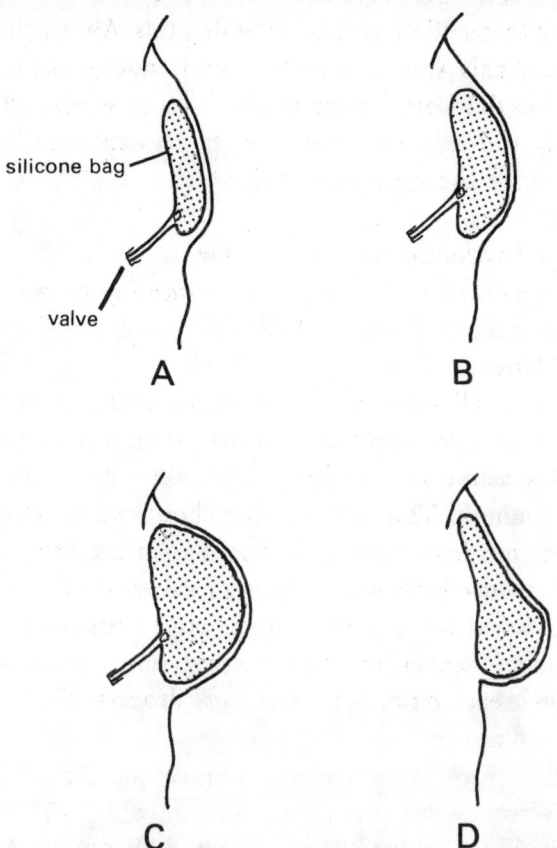

*Fig 7 Tissue expansion.*

control over the expanding shape, and to make a better match with the other breast.

It is sometimes, though not always, unsuitable for women who have had radiotherapy or a radical mastectomy because the skin flaps may be either too thin or too tight to sustain this slow stretching.

## 3. MUSCLE AND SKIN FLAP

These are major operations which use the woman's own body tissue to create the replacement breast. They do sometimes require supplementing with a small silicone implant as well.

'I'm glad I had it done, even though it wasn't easy to go through.'

*Anne*

### Method One (Latissimus Dorsi Myocutaneous Flap) Using Muscle From The Back

A flap of muscle and skin on the back directly behind the operated breast is rotated and pushed through from back to front, and placed on the chest wall. The skin taken from the back supplements what is already on the chest to create an envelope for the muscle which can, if necessary, be bulked out further with a silicone implant placed behind it to match the size of the other breast. The angle and site of the scars are variable and it is important for the woman to decide what is best for her lifestyle. For instance, someone who likes wearing a bikini will want the scar on her back to be as horizontal as possible so that it lies under the bra strap, but another woman who prefers wearing low-backed evening dresses may want to have her scar at an oblique angle and as far to the edge as possible. Round the breast there will be a neat oval scar.

### Method Two (Rectus Abdominus Myocutaneous Flap) Using Muscle From The Abdomen

A flap of muscle and skin taken from the abdominal muscle which runs up from the pubic bone to the breastbone, is rotated and taken up to the breast area. There is usually enough tissue here to match a larger breast without needing an additional silicone implant. Scarring on the abdomen can

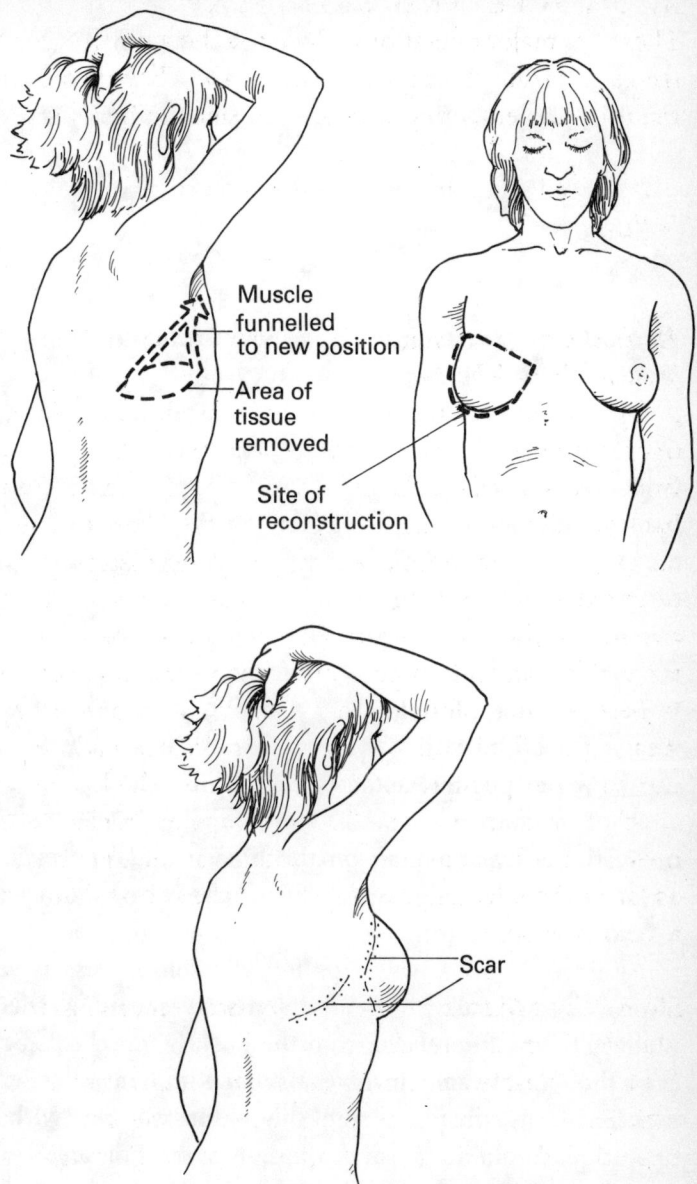

Muscle
funnelled
to new position

Area of
tissue
removed

Site of
reconstruction

Scar

*Fig 8 Breast reconstruction using muscle from the back.*

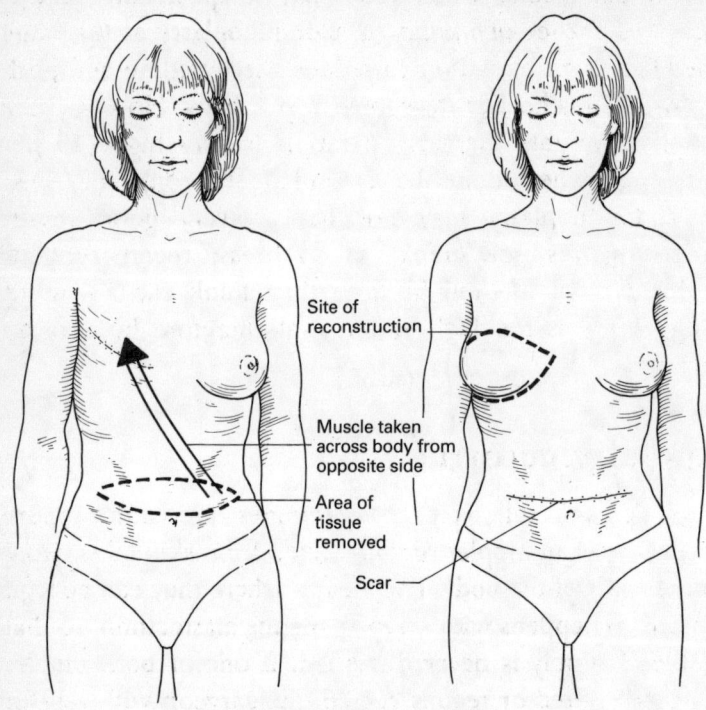

Site of
reconstruction

Muscle taken
across body from
opposite side

Area of
tissue
removed

Scar

*Fig 9 Breast reconstruction using muscle from the abdomen.*

be vertical or horizontal; on the breast it will be oval.

Both these methods are possible for women who have had a radical mastectomy or radiotherapy (or both). The transferred tissue is well supplied with blood vessels which improves the healing process. Generally speaking, the first method using the muscle from the back is more satisfactory, even though it usually involves using an implant as well. Two practised surgeons can combine a mastectomy with this operation in an hour, and there are seldom any serious complications.

Some women, however, are tempted by the second method

because the results, when good, can be spectacular, and it offers the chance of having an abdominoplasty at the same time. This is an operation to reduce the waistline and girth of a woman who has developed a pot belly. However, the complication rate for this operation is very high (45 per cent even when done by a skilled surgeon) and even the abdominoplasty may not have a very good result. Some surgeons now refuse to do breast reconstructions by this second method because they think the risk of it going wrong is too high and that it therefore borders on malpractice.

# Nipple Reconstruction

As a general rule, preserved nipples are much more satisfactory than nipples reconstructed from skin taken from another part of the body. The ideal is where they can be kept in place, as happens with a subcutaneous mastectomy, so that the blood supply is never disturbed. If one or both nipples are to be grafted or reconstructed, the surgeon will wait for a few months before doing the operation to give the breasts time to settle into their permanent position. 'Balancing', as this is called, can pose problems, especially if it's only one nipple which is being replaced. Weight changes, for instance, can seriously skew the result. The reconstructed nipple will usually be made of tissue taken from the healthy nipple, and skin for the areola is taken either from the top of the thigh or the external labia (the lips of the vagina).

Sometimes a nipple or nipples may be grafted onto another part of the body where they are kept until the surgeon is ready to do the breast reconstruction. This can be upsetting, though, if a woman is not fully informed about the procedure as this woman found when she had a bilateral mastectomy followed later by implants.

'The thing I found most difficult to cope with was the fact that my nipples had been grafted to my legs for future replacement. I think perhaps because I hadn't been consulted about this previously, I found this horrific. It was not until about three weeks after the operation that I was even able to look at them or dress them myself.'

*Lesley*

Since the long-term results are so often far from satisfactory, many doctors advise their patients to consider stick-on nipples instead. These can either be moulded to match the existing nipple or they can be bought ready made. Both sorts are effective and the ready-made ones have the additional advantage of being inexpensive. You can buy various biological adhesives from the chemist. One of the most popular is the glue used for sticking on artificial eyelashes.

# 7

## THE HEALING
## PARTNERSHIP

### What Is The Best For Me?

It's difficult to say what is the 'best' treatment for any particular woman, largely because breast cancer is so variable. Surgery of some kind is nearly always advisable, in order to remove the primary tumour in the breast before it starts to spread, but before you consented to your operation the doctor should also have discussed with you the subsequent (adjuvant) treatments he or she thinks you should have. In medical jargon this is called 'managing' the disease; in your terms it's about reviewing all your options and making an informed decision about what you are prepared to accept in the way of treatment.

The three options open to you in orthodox medicine are radiotherapy, chemotherapy and hormone therapy, all of which were briefly described in chapter three. As we saw there, it now seems that there's some quite compelling evidence to show that women with early breast cancer who follow up their initial surgery with a course of either chemotherapy or hormone therapy, (sometimes both) do have a distinctly improved chance of long-term survival. These adjuvant therapies will be presented to you as being a wise precaution to clear up any cancer cells that could be lingering in your body, either in the breast itself or in more distant parts, should some have escaped into the bloodstream or through the lymphatic system. However, they all have side effects, and sometimes these can be quite severe. Because you are seriously ill and you want to get better, you may think side effects, however unpleasant, are relatively unimportant compared to your prime goal of complete recovery from the cancer. All the same, you should be fully aware of what they are and what they could mean to you because, in the same way that the disease is unpredictable, so too can be the results of treatment for it.

Whichever treatment or combination of treatments the doctor proposes, it's done in the belief that it will produce a good result for that particular patient. Sometimes the medical expectation is more than justified; other times, and it could be for no immediately discernible reason, the outcome proves to be disappointing for doctor and patient alike. Your doctor would naturally like to be able to assure you that the treatment is going to work. Since, however, that's not possible, no matter how well-founded the optimism, he or she will do the next best thing and point to all the evidence in its favour.

Some doctors don't keep right up to date with new developments in treatments for breast cancer, and may prefer to stick to what they consider to be a tried and tested procedure. They may be sincerely convinced they are offering their patients the best available treatment, but how can they be so sure if they are not prepared to consider new information? The only way you, the patient, are going to know what kind of doctor is treating you - conservative, open-minded or dogmatic - is by trying to talk through the treatment programme in as detailed a way as possible. If your doctor is not too keen to enter into this kind of dialogue, then it's all the more important to take your time to think carefully about what is being proposed to you. You also need time to talk it over with your family and other people close to you.

Some women may not have surgery at all, but will be offered either radiotherapy or hormone therapy (tamoxifen) instead as their primary treatment. This could be for a variety of reasons. If you are quite elderly, for instance, the doctor may think that surgery would be too much for you, particularly if you are suffering from some other condition such as diabetes. In these circumstances, you will probably be given tamoxifen alone. Or it may be that it is you who has refused surgery; you have asked to start with radiotherapy to see whether the tumour can be successfully removed by that method without losing your breast, but you are prepared to follow up this treatment with chemotherapy or tamoxifen.

The third possibility is that the tumour has become inoperable because it has spread across the chest and may even be ulcerating. This usually happens when a woman has for some reason delayed consulting her doctor or has been persuaded that she is being needlessly anxious. Even in these supposedly more enlightened days, there are still some GPs who will play down a woman's anxiety because they themselves don't understand that it is always important to take any change in the breast seriously. If your cancer is advanced, the doctor will probably advise you that it will be necessary to start with chemotherapy in an effort to shrink the tumour.

'I had this indentation as if something were drawing the breast in, but he told me it was just my age and not to worry. So I went away and left it for another year, but it was getting worse all the time so I went back to him and this time I insisted he send me to a specialist.'

*Fern (then 40)*

Never agree to 'wait and see'. You may be reading this book because you are worried about your breast health or know someone else who is. Any concern at all should be reported immediately to your doctor, and if there is any doubt in your mind about his or her opinion, don't be afraid to ask for a referral to a specialist. Nine out of ten breast lumps turn out to be harmless, which is reassuring for most of us. All the same there is a crucial difference between knowing the truth and worrying about what you don't know. Even if you are unlucky and the truth in your case turns out not to be good news, you may still find it preferable to deal with the devil you know than the phantom you fear.

It wouldn't be surprising if, after having been presented with a variety of options for treatment, you end up feeling somewhat confused but pretty sure that you would like to have another opinion. Since cancer treatment in general tends so often to be based on a doctor's personal preference, it will certainly do no harm for you to seek out another professional point of view. Even if the new doctor doesn't tell you anything very different from the first doctor, at least you will have the satisfaction of knowing that you have explored an alternative approach. It will be less necessary for you to do this if you are being treated in a cancer centre where the specialists work together as a team and jointly discuss and plan the treatment for each patient. Even here, however, in a milieu where experience and knowledge are pooled there will be clashes of opinion.

X treatment may work for Y number of women and promise them Z number of extra years, but what sometimes gets left out of these equations is that what we are talking about is people, not statistics. You have to weigh up the risks and benefits as you see them for yourself. Medical reports of 'successful' new treatments, which are sometimes no more than a new cocktail of the same anti-cancer drugs, tend to skate over the side effects. Patients are described as either more or less 'compliant', but what this really means is that some patients are less able, or less willing than others to tolerate the nausea and vomiting accompanying, for instance, chemotherapy. This is not because they are morally feeble but because their bodies react differently.

They may also have strong views about what they are and aren't prepared to accept, particularly since no honest doctor can swear, hand on heart, that any of these treatments actually saves lives. They prolong them, possibly, but then you have to ask: at what cost? That is a question doctors find very hard to answer. In the end, each individual patient has to find the answer for herself.

An interesting study has shown that many people when diagnosed with cancer, an illness they rightly perceive as life-threatening, are often desperately eager to accept highly toxic treatment, however slight the benefit, if they think it offers them a chance. By comparison, oncologists, cancer nurses and members of the general public who were asked the same basic questions: namely, would they accept intensive or mild treatments of chemotherapy which offered them very reduced effectiveness - no more than 1 per cent chance of cure or relief of symptoms and life prolonged by only three months - were much more dubious. Among the doctors, it is interesting to note that the radiotherapists were the least enthusiastic of all.

The study isn't representative of the whole patient population, because it excludes those people who had already opted out by dint of refusing any chemotherapy at all. Doctors will say that in practice few patients do decline the opportunity of this or any other treatment, but there are no figures available; nor do we have any idea how many more drop out at a later stage because they find the treatment unbearable.

Obviously, the dosage and particular combination of drugs are important but even so, doctors are often surprised that one patient has such a bad reaction while another emerges comparatively unscathed. Here are the experiences of two women, both in their thirties and both with early breast cancer who were given very similar treatments: a lumpectomy followed by radiotherapy and chemotherapy.

'After the operation I felt pleased to have survived and that the worst was over. I felt I could face up to any other treatment. The radiotherapy lasted for six weeks and it made me feel tired and a bit sick so I gave up working. I couldn't cope with the chemotherapy. The injections took ten minutes. It was awful stuff. I'm not really sure that it does any good. I stopped after three injections and now I'm on tamoxifen - half dose because the full dose gave me terrible hot flushes and I put on weight.'

*Katrina*

'I recovered very quickly from the op. I came in every day for the radiotherapy. The radiologist was not very good at handling women with breast cancer. He was blunt and tactless so I refused to talk to him. Then I had chemotherapy. I was amazed how little it affected me. I didn't lose my hair. I didn't feel sick and I was able to go straight off on a skiing holiday.'

*Vera*

# Adjuvant Therapies – What To Expect

## RADIOTHERAPY

### *External*

After your operation the radiotherapist will draw up a treatment plan for you, which is precisely tailored to deal with your particular type of tumour and where it is situated in the breast. Careful planning is a vital preliminary to radiotherapy, because it is crucial to deliver a very precise dosage (the minimum effective dose) and to target it exactly. The radiotherapist will explain what is involved and you will then be taken to the simulator unit where the radiographer will measure the area to be radiated, and draw lines on your skin with indelible ink to outline it. You may also have some X-rays taken to help define the area.

All this takes a bit of time (possibly an hour, and occasionally a repeat visit may be necessary before the radiotherapist is absolutely happy that the plan is right). It means lying still on your back having first had your arm and hand on the side to be treated carefully positioned. This can be rather uncomfortable so soon after the operation, but you can take comfort from the thought that when you have your actual treatment it will be far quicker - quite literally only a few minutes - and the entire session, including undressing and dressing again, may take no more than half an hour. Wear tops with skirts or trousers rather than dresses because you only need to strip to the waist. You will also be expected to remove any jewellery.

You will be receiving this treatment every day for four to six weeks and the appointment will usually be at the same time every day so that you can establish a routine. It also gives you 24 hours of recovery time. All the same, the travelling and the effect of the treatment will take its toll (see below) so you will probably find it helps to take, if you can, a short rest every day, or at the very least slow up your life a bit, especially if you have a family to look after or have gone back to work.

'I insisted on driving myself to the treatment. I found it very sociable - like going to a club.'

*Sue*

### Side Effects

They vary quite considerably and while some unlucky people seem to get them all, others may feel pretty good all the way through. It's quite likely, however, that you will feel tired and possibly a bit queasy. Some people also get low and depressed and generally lose their appetite for life. Weight loss is also quite common. Others, though feeling quite well in themselves, may instead have to cope with a strong skin reaction.

'It made no difference that I've got a black skin. It just got blacker and hurt a lot, but it's all right now.'

*Una*

Some skin reaction with radiotherapy is inevitable, and much depends on the type of skin you have and your age. Before you start your treatment, the radiotherapist will advise you about skin care and probably also give you a booklet to take home. At best, the reaction will be rather like an acute case of sunburn, becoming red and quite painful. If it shows signs of soreness or 'weeping', the radiographer will suggest some cream for it. Keep your clothing loose and free round the treated area, and it's probably best to do without a bra if that doesn't make you too uncomfortable.

The radiographer will give you very detailed advice about skin care which it's essential to follow. If you have any problems let her know immediately. Here are some basic guidelines:

1. Don't let the treated area get wet, so be especially careful in your bath.
2. Bathe any skin near to the treated area in tepid water and pat dry with a soft towel.
3. Don't apply any deodorant or scented talcum powder to

the treated area. Baby powder should be all right, but check first with the radiographer.

4. Don't rub or scratch the treated area.
5. Don't shave your armpit. If that area is being radiated you will lose hair from there, permanently, but not from anywhere else on your body.
6. Wear loose garments on your top half, preferably made of natural fibres like cotton or silk, especially where they are in contact with your skin.
7. Keep the treated skin out of sunlight for at least a year, possibly longer.

There are also some long-term side effects of which you should be aware. Unfortunately, they sometimes don't get mentioned until they happen!

### Change in Skin Texture

The irradiated skin may change its texture, feeling thicker and less sensitive. If you had a lumpectomy only, your breast may become firmer and harder. Sometimes it shrinks a bit and changes colour, but this is usually only in cases where radiotherapy was administered many years ago when doses tended to be higher and less carefully targeted.

### Swollen Arm

You may develop puffiness in your arm and hand on the treated side. This is because either radiotherapy or surgery (or both) have destroyed the lymph nodes under the arm. This means that the lymphatic fluid can no longer drain away, and it can result in a long-term condition called lymphoedema, which requires early skilled treatment otherwise it will become troublesome and painful. Don't delay if you have any problems. Should your GP or consultant (or both) be unsympathetic, it's advisable to go to a specialist lymphoedema clinic (see Useful Addresses). For more information about treatments for lymphoedema see chapter eight.

Meanwhile, here are some basic precautions you should adopt permanently to protect your hand and arm so as to prevent this condition occurring:

1. Always offer the arm on the untreated side for blood pressure testing or sampling; the same applies for vaccinations or injections.
2. Protect the arm and hand on the treated side from cuts, burns, grazes etc. by wearing gloves for chores and gardening.
3. Wear long sleeves in the summer to protect against sunburn.
4. Wear a thimble for sewing.
5. Keep up the exercises you first learnt in hospital (see chapter eight).

*Increased Risk of Heart Disease*

If your left breast has been irradiated there is a possibility that the heart arteries may be damaged by the radiation. A recent study has shown that this can happen, causing them to narrow over time, particularly in cases where women were treated some years ago when the radiation dose was so much higher. If you have had radiotherapy for cancer in your left breast and are, therefore, now feeling understandably anxious, I would suggest you ask your GP to refer you to a cardiologist for a check-up. You will probably be perfectly all right, but should something be wrong, you can receive treatment before the condition worsens. If you are now about to have treatment in the left breast, you should ask the radiotherapist to make sure your heart is screened, if at all possible, by a shield to protect it from radiation.

*Internal*

One thing you can feel reassured about is that if you have external radiation you won't become radioactive. In the case of internal radiation (described on page 47) you will be radioactive for the time during which you are having treatment, but since this will only be for a few days while you are in hospital, it isn't too daunting a prospect. It means spending quite a lot of your time on your own, and visitors will be restricted. Pregnant women and children will not be allowed to see you at all and you will be cared for in a separate room off the ward.

> 'I was so lucky to be in a hospital where they were offering this treatment. It was a bit scary to have radioactive wires threaded through my breast but it's all been worth it. I think more women should be told about it.'
>
> *Janice*

## CHEMOTHERAPY

Like radiotherapy, this is a treatment which requires planning. From the time the cancer is diagnosed your doctors will have a good idea of what drugs they think you will need and indeed, may start you on them before surgery. Until very recently, many doctors thought that chemotherapy for early breast cancer was more effective in younger women who had not yet had the menopause. Now, however, as revealed in the *Lancet* report mentioned in chapter three, the evidence suggests that a course of chemotherapy plus tamoxifen may significantly improve the outlook for many older women as well.

Chemotherapy is most usually given by mouth (tablets), by injection or intravenously, which means it comes through a drip. Doctors like to start the first course as soon as possible after surgery and some doctors use a 'cold cap' as a way of reducing hair loss. This is an ice cold cap which the woman wears during treatment. Its effect is temporarily to narrow the blood vessels on the scalp, thus decreasing the amount of chemotherapy which can penetrate into the hair follicles. It works only with certain drugs. If the chemotherapy is to be administered by injection or intravenously, this usually involves a short stay in hospital. Sometimes it is done on an out-patient basis, but more usually you will be admitted overnight.

Each course and combination of drugs is individually tailored and may be modified from time to time. This explains why one woman may have chemotherapy over three months, and another over six months or longer, sometimes on a weekly basis, sometimes monthly. Some courses are much more toxic than others. Your doctor will know the likely side effects you will suffer and it's important to discuss them beforehand. They include:

1. Extreme nausea and vomiting
2. Constipation or diarrhoea
3. Partial or total hair loss from head and body but it does grow back, sometimes thicker and slightly curly
4. Mouth ulcers
5. Fatigue
6. Vulnerability to infection
7. Depression
8. Loss of sexual interest and libido.

These are the most common ones, but there are others and you should report anything unusual to your doctor. BACUP has a helpful booklet on chemotherapy which has sensible tips for dealing with physical problems like extreme nausea and unremitting vomiting. However, advice to drink plenty of fluid and avoid fatty foods is no more than common sense and it may not prove sufficient to cope entirely with this or other side effects. At the end of this chapter we suggest some alternative approaches.

The emotional and psychological problems that may be induced by chemotherapy can be quite as difficult to handle. It isn't really very reassuring to be told you will feel better again when the treatment stops. For you as for many others, it is precisely during your treatment that you particularly want all the support and understanding you can find. Sexual problems like loss of libido and an inability to reach orgasm may cause problems in a formerly happy sexual relationship. If this is now to be denied to you, life may become dismal and lonely indeed. It may also explain why many women give up on their chemotherapy: it introduces just one problem too many at a time when living is quite hard enough.

'The chemo was awful – as if I was having terrible morning sickness. I couldn't even listen to the radio, but as time went on during the five months the treatment lasted I did find ways within myself of handling it better, and I felt I wanted to help others through this difficult time – most of the women the BCMA ask me to talk to are having chemotherapy.'

*Sue*

## HORMONE THERAPY

### Tamoxifen

This is the generic name for a synthetic anti-oestrogen hormone which is today the most popular treatment for breast cancer. Although the exact process is not understood, it appears to work by blocking the supply of oestrogen, the hormone which is undoubtedly implicated in most breast cancers. Doctors are happy to prescribe this anti-oestrogen, taken in tablet form, because they know it's effective and it also has relatively low toxicity. Even if they can't promise a cure with it, they can say with confidence that it appears to prolong, often by several years, a period of disease-free life. It has a very high success rate for preventing cancer occurring in the other breast, and it is also used to deal with a recurrence of cancer.

The side effects it does produce are usually described by doctors as 'minor' and 'short-term'. For many women this may be true, and they may be prepared to put up with hot flushes, weight gain, and menstrual upsets (if they are pre-menopausal), because they believe the benefits far outweigh the disadvantages. Unfortunately, some doctors go so overboard in their enthusiasm for this treatment that they assure their patients that tamoxifen has no side effects at all. This is simply not true. An active drug by its very nature must produce a reaction of some kind, and to pretend otherwise does neither the patient nor the doctor any good. It could also be dangerous, because a woman told she need not expect side effects will think she must be imagining her symptoms, and hesitate to report them to her doctor for fear of being thought a hypochondriac or a fantasist.

Furthermore, since tamoxifen has only been in use for a relatively short time (since the mid-seventies) we can't yet be certain that it won't have delayed and possibly more serious side effects. A Swedish study where the dose was 40 mg a day (higher than normally given in this country) found an increase in cases of endometrial cancer (lining of the womb). Although this cancer can be treated and usually cured if picked up in the early stages, it's hardly desirable that in the process of being treated for one cancer a woman is induced to have another. Another rare but serious complication which has been reported more than once is retinopathy, which can lead to irreversible blindness. There is also some concern that tamoxifen may produce tumours in the liver. Trials have shown that it does in rats and although rats metabolize the drug differently from humans, the question has not yet been fully answered. On the positive side, it seems that tamoxifen could have a preventive effect for heart disease, as it appears to lower cholesterol levels, and also for osteoporosis.

Tamoxifen has been used in three million women, and it has given relief and a hope of reprieve to many. Two years seems to be the minimum period of time for an effective dosage. No one yet knows whether longer - five years for example - also means better. Side effects that might occur and should be reported to your doctor include:

1. Unexpected vaginal bleeding
2. Blurred vision/headaches
3. Menstrual changes of any sort - irregular periods, no periods or painful periods
4. Dry vagina
5. Vaginal discharge
6. Hot flushes
7. Weight gain
8. Growth of facial hair, changes in skin texture
9. Voice deepening
10. Aches and pains of any sort

### Ovarian Ablation

The ovaries can be removed by surgery or irradiated by radiotherapy. Sometimes chemotherapy will have the same effect. With all these treatments, the ovaries are put out of action permanently so that you will no longer ovulate and an artificial menopause is induced. This means you will not be able to have children.

Doctors (usually male) sometimes find it hard to understand why a woman in her mid to late thirties or forties, facing a life-threatening disease, should grieve for her loss of fertility, especially if she already has a family. To them it may seem an irrelevant side issue when compared with the gravity of her cancer, but for the woman in question the reality may be quite different.

Her cancer frightens her. She has probably had to accept surgery which makes her feel mutilated, no matter how carefully it is performed, and sometimes the scar is needlessly ugly. Now she is being asked to relinquish her fertility as well. It is more than the ability to reproduce; her fertility is symbolic of her womanhood, and it seems like one sacrifice too many. Of course it is distressing. Ask any man how he would feel if he had to lose his fertility! And for a woman who has never had children, the loss may be more poignant still. She grieves in the knowledge that her chance to have them has gone for ever. Her regret is now exacerbated by the unpleasant symptoms invading her that tend always to be stronger when the menopause is artificially induced: hot flushes, dry vagina, pain during intercourse, dry hair and skin, panic attacks and so on are all possible.

Offering HRT as a compensation may not always appear the ideal solution doctors would like it to be, quite apart from the fact that its possible link with some cases of breast cancer has not yet been ruled out.

## Staying Whole

The orthodox treatments described above (in particular radiotherapy and chemotherapy) work in a fairly crude way by attacking and destroying the cancer cells. In the process, healthy cells in the vicinity of the tumour will also be affected. In due course, when the treatment is over, the damaged tissue will mostly recover, but while it's going on you may feel mentally in low spirits and physically drained by the side effects. It's hardly surprising, since your immune system is being knocked out by a massive assault and you may be having to cope with other problems in your life, some perhaps caused by your illness. It's a cruel paradox that just at the time when you need to feel at your strongest and best, your state of health is being undermined in order to cure you.

This is not invariably the case, and some women sail through their treatment, almost exhilarated by it because they feel the end result will be worth it all. But their sense of let-down may come later. As we saw in chapter five, many women become depressed when they return home or when the treatment is finished. They've no longer got an obvious objective to fight for and now they're on their own.

Conventional (orthodox) treatments in cancer focus on the particular diseased part of your body. It may require more than one type of treatment, but basically the intention remains the same: an all-out effort is concentrated on removing malignant tissue and preventing spread into other parts of the body. A caring, holistically-minded doctor will try to make this unpleasant process as humane as possible, but it's not easy. These treatments take their toll, and not only of patients. Those who care for cancer patients cannot fail to be affected by the pain and suffering they see every day, especially as much of it is inflicted by the treatments they believe in but can't guarantee.

They tend to react in one of three ways. They may distance themselves, and seek to justify their detachment by throwing their energy behind some separate but related activity like cancer research where they can reassure themselves that they are working for a worthy goal. Alternatively, they may cut themselves off completely from what they see and hear around them, sometimes developing an apparently cold and indifferent carapace, which explains why some patients have such distressing encounters with their doctors. Finally, there are those with a genuinely holistic attitude, who are concerned about all aspects of patient welfare and this leads them to encourage their patients to seek support and comfort from wherever they can find it. Holistic doctors realize that orthodox cancer medicine, particularly as epitomized by many of the modern 'brutalist' treatments, while successful in many cases, is, nonetheless, the antithesis of all that is meant by 'whole-person' medicine. It can't and doesn't pretend to treat the whole person – mind and spirit as well as body. However, there is a growing recognition, even among the more conservative oncologists, that many of their patients need psychological help for problems that often arise as a direct result of their treatments. Breast care nurse counsellors have an important part to play here.

> 'I feel like the manager of a pea canning factory. I have 3,000 people coming through the door every year for radiotherapy and chemotherapy and some of it's pretty dreadful. They can't miss their slot because we run a production line, but anything that helps them support better what's being done to them and gain more benefit from their treatment can only be good as far as I'm concerned.'
>
> *Professor Karol Sikora, Hammersmith Hospital, London*

Professor Sikora, who sees himself as essentially a pragmatist plucking the best available for his patients from all quarters, is pioneering a radically different approach to cancer treatment. Firmly mainstream in his own specialty as a cancer physician, he has no qualms about broadening the range of treatment options beyond the conventional limits. A few years ago he invited Penny Brohn and her team from the Bristol Cancer Help Centre to help him incorporate some of the better-known complementary therapies into his wards.

Pleased with the results, he is now well on the way to achieving his appeal target for £5 million to create the Hammersmith Cancer Centre which should be fully functional by 1995 at the latest.

The building is already in progress and design features are planned which are more usually associated with a luxury hotel. There will be a central atrium, internal fountains, a real coffee shop in place of the familiar dreary rows of plastic seats serviced by a drinks machine, and full length glass walls in the wards overlooking planted terraces. The stated aim is to 'provide an environment where patient comfort and support have a clear priority, where patients are involved as far as possible with decisions about treatment options, and where the research and specialist resources are available on site to ensure that the presented options can always give the full benefits of current medical knowledge.' Complementary therapies will be offered to all patients alongside the conventional treatments.

Professor Sikora already operates a day care centre, managed by three oncology nurses who are in charge of coordinating and administering all the treatments. He maintains 'they do it much better than most doctors', and they work together with the supportive care manager who coordinates all the complementary therapists. Massage, aromatherapy, relaxation, reflexology, visualization, homoeopathy, healing, group therapy and counselling are just some of the treatments on offer. In the new unit the day care centre is envisaged as the hub of the whole operation: it will be 'a sympathetic meeting place' for patients, medical staff and therapists where they will be able to discuss treatments as well as receive and give them. The welcoming atmosphere should banish the sense of fear and the isolation that so many patients suffer when they have to attend hospital for adjuvant therapy.

It's a great concept – what Professor Sikora calls 'building a patient's will to survive' – and when it's all in place the Hammersmith Cancer Centre will provide a marvellous example of the healing partnership that can and should exist between conventional and complementary treatments. It shows that instead of being antagonistic and mutually suspicious of each other's motivation, which usually means that the hapless patient ends up as piggy in the middle, not knowing who to heed or where to turn, therapists from both ends of the spectrum can, with good will, work together for the patient's benefit. This is holism in action.

The Hammersmith is not the only hospital to encourage complementary therapies. The Royal Marsden, the famous cancer hospital in London, also offers a wide range. 'Anything a patient wants we will try to give them – special diets, art therapy,' says Richard Wells, head of the rehabilitation unit there. St Bartholomew's Hospital in the City of London is another, and there are several hospitals up and down the UK where the consultants are sufficiently open-minded to allow a few complementary therapists on their wards. Spiritual healing, for instance, has been available in many NHS wards for a long time. Often it is an enterprising nurse who has become interested in a therapeutic skill like massage or aromatherapy, and taken a training course, who will suggest that she offer it to patients. If you want to continue with a particular therapy while you are in hospital or are interested in starting something you have been recommended, it's advisable to tell your consultant, as tactfully as possible, that you would like your therapist to visit you on the ward.

All this is an amazing advance on even five years ago, when it would have been unthinkable to have anyone but strictly orthodox medical staff in the wards. This is, of course, still the situation in the majority of hospitals, so that most patients will have to make their own arrangements, and pay for them out of their own pockets, if they want some form of complementary therapy. Some people may prefer this because it leaves them completely free to make their own choice. Professor Sikora is concerned that in these budget-conscious times, when every hospital has to cost out in detail everything it does, support services like these may be dropped since their benefits can't be quantified in the obvious way that you can cost many surgical procedures. Yet the cost of complementary medicine is low. In Professor Sikora's unit, where the whole department costs £3.8 million a year to run, the complementary medicine services account for a mere £40,000.

## The 'Feel Good' Factor

Professor Sikora admits that he has no idea how the complementary therapies work, but then that is equally true of many drugs. The only thing that concerns him is the effect any treatment has on the patient, but he does allow himself to speculate whether a treatment which succeeds in modifying stress may not also sometimes modify the tumour, at least temporarily.

There is one interesting scientific study giving some support for this hypothesis, where two matched groups of patients with advanced breast cancer were either offered an active weekly programme of group therapy and self-hypnosis to control pain, or nothing. The latter control group fared half as well as those who had group therapy. David Spiegel and his fellow researchers are careful to emphasize that those in the intervention group were never encouraged to believe either that the therapy would cure them, or that if they developed the right mental attitude they could overcome their disease. 'The emphasis in our programme was on living as fully as possible, improving communication with family members and doctors, facing and mastering fears about death and dying, and controlling pain and other symptoms.'

The major outstanding difference between complementary therapies and orthodox cancer treatments is that the latter usually make you feel rotten and frequently cause other conditions which also need treatment (the iatrogenic effect, meaning medically induced illness), whereas complementary treatments usually have the reverse effect. They tend to make you feel better in yourself, less stressed, more able to cope with your treatments and your problems; in short, it's the 'feel good' factor at work. These gentle treatments may not cure you, they may not even do you any good that can be positively attributed to them, like reversing tumour growth, for example, but they do make you feel better and that, for any cancer patient, can be priceless.

Of course, there are exceptions on both sides, but let me anticipate the opposition before it starts shouting. Yes, some women find their orthodox treatments are relatively non-traumatic and feel no need for any supplementary support. Yes, there are a few gruelling, usually frankly cranky alternative treatments which make patients feel sick, depressed and sometimes deeply guilty, either because they have not been able to persist with them, or because they have been told their cancer is their fault. Certainly there are some dangerous and dogmatic alternative practitioners around who will take merciless advantage of a cancer sufferer's desperation. They will insist that all orthodox medicine is bad for you and that you must follow their regimen exclusively, usually at great expense, emotional and monetary, to you.

But just how different is such an unscrupulous person from the hospital consultant who will storm at a patient who has confided that she would like to have some complementary therapy, and possibly even threaten to stop treating her? Or the doctor who presents a particular treatment to a patient as being the one appropriate for their condition, when in fact it is part of a trial into which the patient has been randomly entered without her knowledge and therefore without her informed consent?

When a study funded by the Cancer Research Campaign appeared to show that women who attended the Bristol Cancer Help Centre did significantly less well than those attending NHS hospitals solely for orthodox treatments, the unsavoury glee expressed in some medical circles was moderated not at all by the same people expressing hypocritical regrets that women should have been so gullible as to swallow the 'vile diet' along with the other 'fads'. It wasn't long before the study was exposed as seriously flawed, both in its design and the conclusions it drew. Suddenly most of the names on the paper published in the *Lancet* seemed to have vanished (one committed suicide) and no-one today among the medical researchers has been willing to take responsibility for the distress they have caused, in particular to the many survivors of the study who have now formed their own pressure group to try and obtain an official retraction. Meanwhile the Bristol centre has lost many of its staff and most of its clients and with great difficulty, even at the time of writing, is hauling itself back from the brink of bankruptcy.

Cancer patients don't need anyone to give them sermons about what is or is not 'good' for them. What they do need is advice and information to help them find that elusive 'feel good' factor which will enable them to feel stronger and better able to cope with their disease. There is not the space in this book to write at any length about all the beneficial complementary therapies which are available, but the extensive bibliography and resources section at the end should help you in your search. A book I would particularly recommend is *How To Be a Healthy Patient* by Stephen Fulder which has a chapter devoted to treatments, both psychological and physical, to help cancer patients going through radiotherapy and chemotherapy get the best from their conventional treatments and overcome side effects.

Vitamin supplementation is advisable at least a week before you start any of the hospital treatments, and a change to a naturopathic diet, which involves eating many more raw and unprocessed foods than you are probably used to, could help counteract the acute toxicity induced by drugs. This does, however, involve quite a lot of effort on your part, squeezing juices and finding the suppliers with the right foods. For some people this is a challenge they relish, because it makes them feel they are really contributing to their own recovery. Others may find it too much and will want more help and support, particularly in the early stages, such as can be obtained from a medical herbalist or a homoeopathic doctor. Ginseng is particularly recommended for dealing with stress. Apart from the various meditation and relaxation techniques already mentioned in chapter four, you could consider hypnotherapy or acupuncture to help you overcome side effects like nausea or vomiting from chemotherapy, sometimes so extreme that a patient only has to think of the ward or the nurse who gives her the injection to be sick. The hospital will probably offer you an anti-emetic drug, but you may prefer the idea of harnessing your own mental energies to overcome the problem.

This, indeed, is the whole point of all these therapies. They enable you to regain some control of the situation because you decide how you want to help yourself. The good complementary therapist will offer you sympathy and comfort, sometimes in a very direct way through the hands-on technique of the therapy itself, sometimes simply by listening. Such therapies are empowering in a physical sense because they enable you to rekindle the powers of self-healing we all have within us. They treat the whole person – body, mind and spirit – and even if they don't finally cure you, they will certainly have a restorative effect and make you feel better in yourself and more able to live your life fully.

'Self-help is the essence of complementary therapy. Going to Bristol was the answer to the question I had asked myself – what can I do? We could try out anything we liked, but it was the support and love in the place which was wonderful. It gave me the time to be a cancer bore and chat endlessly about myself with other people who did the same with me.'

*Heather*

# 8

## *LOOKING GOOD*

### From Inside Out

When you are still in hospital but thinking about your return home, one of the concerns uppermost in your mind will undoubtedly be your appearance. Dressed or undressed, whether you have had a total or partial mastectomy, or, alternatively, a breast reconstruction, you will be understandably anxious about how you are going to look - to yourself, to your partner, to your children and to the world in general. Most women, whatever their age, like to look their best - not necessarily glossy glamour girl looks, but simply feeling comfortable with the image they present. The older we get, the more likely we are to feel settled about the way we look and the style we have evolved, and this is the way we want to go on looking.

The majority of women with breast cancer in the UK still have a mastectomy, and most of them want to replace the breast that has been removed with a breast form called a prosthesis. Gone are the days, thank goodness, when a woman had to accept a misshapen bag containing birdseed or lentils (literally!) and stuff it into her bra, hoping she wouldn't rustle too audibly. Today, there is an excellent range of both prostheses and specially cut mastectomy bras to fit every shape, colour and size of woman.

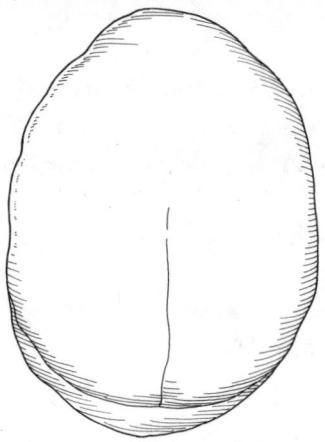

*Fig 10 The Cumfie.*

Some women decide they would prefer to do without a prosthesis, or that they will only wear one when they go out. This is an easier decision to make if you are small-breasted, but for the woman with large and heavy breasts a prosthesis may be essential. Without it she would feel extremely uncomfortable and lopsided. You will have plenty of time to make up your mind what you do want, because for the first weeks after surgery you can wear only a very lightweight prosthesis which restores your shape but doesn't press on the scar and tender area around it. You can also wear this at night inside a sleep bra.

There are several kinds of lightweight prosthesis available for these early days and you will be given one to wear in hospital, but if you don't like it for some reason you might like to contact the BCMA who supply their own version called a Cumfie at cost price (currently £2.50 including postage and packing) in the following cup sizes: AAA, AA, A, B, C, D, DD. Betty Westgate designed the Cumfie many years ago when she realized that nothing suitably lightweight and non-irritant was available for these immediately post-operative weeks. It is made of a washable fabric and is filled with fluffy acrylic fibre which can be washed and spin-dried in a washing machine. Even today she and her husband continue to produce Cumfies in large quantities, making them at home and supplying them to the BCMA.

The filler inside the Cumfie has other uses. If you have had a lumpectomy where relatively little breast tissue has been removed, or a breast reconstruction which has left your new breast imperfectly matched to the other one, you may like to make your own tiny Cumfie pad and sew it into your bra to cover the indentation. Or you can just use a bit of loose Cumfie filler and stuff it into your bra in the place where there is a gap. Another solution is to buy a padded bra and remove the padding from the normal side so that the two breasts match up.

Once the soreness has worn off and the scar has healed – usually about six to eight weeks after surgery, or a little longer if you have been having radiotherapy – you will be ready to make an appointment to be fitted for your permanent prosthesis. The hospital Appliance Officer will probably visit you in the out-patients clinic although sometimes she (alas, occasionally it's a 'he') will make a preliminary visit to measure you and discuss your requirements while you are still in the ward.

## Choosing A Prosthesis

The modern prosthesis is made from a silicone material which warms to the body temperature, feels soft like skin, comes in various tints to match your own skin colour and moves like a real breast. It comes with or without a moulded nipple, or you can get a separate stick-on nipple to match your real one.

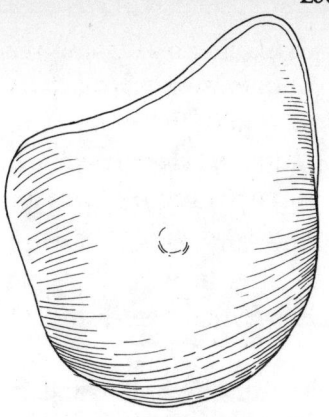

**Fig 11  Full prosthesis.**

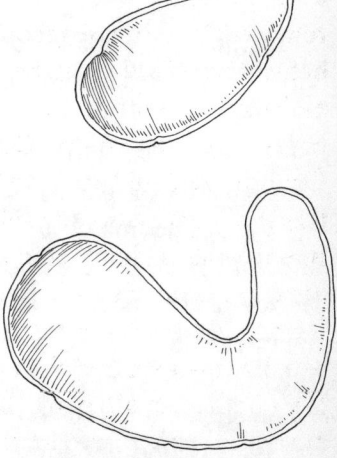

**Fig 12  Partial prostheses.**

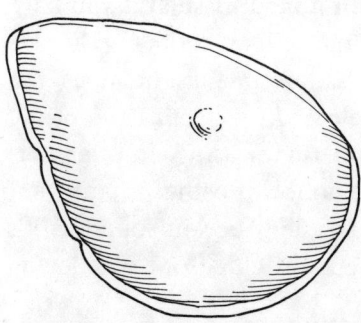

**Fig 13  Shell prosthesis.**

It has a polyurethane outer skin which is quite impermeable so that you can safely swim in the sea or swimming pool without fear that it will either absorb water like a sponge or become damaged by the salt or chlorine. Most prostheses are supplied with one or two washable cotton covers which make them more comfortable to wear, especially in hot weather, and they can either be slipped inside an ordinary bra or held inside an internal pocket in the bra cup (rather like absorbent pads for nursing mothers).

Prostheses are made for the right and left breast and in shapes that are adapted for the particular operation you may have had. There are also partial prostheses made in the same silicone material, and available in various shapes to fit women who have had a partial mastectomy and want to round out their shape to match the other breast. The shell prosthesis offers an alternative way of concealing a partial mastectomy. Hollow at the back, it slips over the breast which has been operated on, the extra layer filling it out and concealing any indentations.

The shell prosthesis combined with an interior stabilizing pad is also a godsend for the woman who has a naturally heavy bust, because it's lighter than the full breast form and, therefore, more comfortable to wear. (Silicone, lifelike though it is in many ways, is heavier than human tissue.) If you have very large breasts, your surgeon may suggest reducing the size of your healthy breast at the same time as he does the mastectomy. Many women are pleased to accept this option. And finally, here's one more handy tip for using Cumfie filler: as a lightweight stuffing behind a hollow prosthesis to prevent any chance of making an embarrassing suction sound as it's released from pressure, say, when you come out of a loving clinch.

Most of these prostheses are available free on the National Health Service, so in theory every woman should get the prosthesis that suits her best. Unfortunately, this happens far less often than it should, because purchasing policy varies between the different health authorities and you may be shown a restricted range simply because the Appliance Officer's budget does not stretch to more than two or three types of prosthesis.

There are other shortcomings about the service. You may be given an appointment for fitting many weeks after the operation, whereas what you want is to be able to wear the prosthesis as soon as the tenderness has worn off. The hospital fitting room is often no more than a dingy boxroom, filled to overflowing with trusses, false limbs and corsets, with no room to turn around, and sometimes it even lacks a mirror, an obvious essential for good fitting. The fitter's attitude can also leave much to be desired - offhand, unsympathetic or giving the impression that time, rather than the client, is the top priority. Male fitters can be unbearably jovial, no doubt to hide their embarrassment. Most of them would prefer not to be doing this particular job, as they recognize how inappropriate it is for a man.

## Fitting A Prosthesis

If you are encountering problems of this kind at your hospital, one way of getting round them is to book a free appointment with a BCMA fitter at the Association's headquarters in London. Here you will be given privacy, comfort and an uninterrupted hour to discuss your needs with a woman who is an expert at her job and brings experience and empathy to it. The BCMA holds a large stock of prostheses, bras and swimwear which is constantly updated. The fitter can show you the entire range of prostheses available under the NHS plus others, and although you can't buy anything from the

BCMA itself, she will be able to tell you where you can find whatever has taken your fancy.

The BCMA keeps a comprehensive and regularly updated list of stockists and mail order firms supplying prostheses and specially designed bras, lingerie and beachwear. This stock list is available on request free of charge. The BCMA can also give you the name of a specialist mastectomy fitting and advisory service in your area if London is too far to come. The advantage of the BCMA fitting service is that it takes no commission from any manufacturer so you can be sure the advice you receive will be unbiased and geared entirely to meeting your individual needs.

For your fitting, whether you go to the BCMA or elsewhere, you should bring with you a couple of bras and some favourite tops. But don't be surprised if the first thing the fitter suggests to you is to try on a slightly larger bra. Apparently, this is the great British failing – we are all spilling out of bras that are one, if not more sizes too small. You might also like to bring with you a low-necked dress so that you can see how you will look on different occasions. Incidentally, it's most unwise to throw out any of your clothes before you have had this fitting, because you may be pleasantly surprised at how easy it is to do a few simple adaptations and keep them all. It's important that one of the tops you bring should be quite tight-fitting so that you can look at yourself from every angle in the mirrors and be sure that the prosthesis and bra together give you a good smooth outline.

If your fitting is at the BCMA, once you have made your choice of prosthesis, the fitter will write down on headed BCMA paper your exact requirements – the name, number and description of the model and the manufacturer. This you can take back to the hospital appliance fitter and ask to have it ordered for you. This free NHS service is continued indefinitely. All you have to do when your prosthesis begins to show signs of wear and tear (probably after two to three years) is to ask the consultant at the hospital where you go for your check-ups to sign a prescription form for you, preferably worded 'prosthesis to suit'. You may need to get a new prosthesis if you find that you change breast size, due to putting on or losing weight, or because of the medication you are taking. If you need another prosthesis for this or any other reason you are, of course, entitled to have it free of charge.

Should you move to another part of the country, or if it is some years since your operation and you no longer go for check-ups, you can ask your GP to send a note to a consultant at the local hospital who will give you a new prescription. It should have the same wording as before, and you should make sure that your GP includes the following details in his or her letter: your name and address, the date of your mastectomy, and whether it's partial or total. The surgeon can send the prescription either to your doctor or directly to you, and you can then make an appointment either with the Appliance Officer at the hospital or an approved NHS stockist and fitter. It's always worth looking at the range available rather than just re-ordering what you had before, because the prosthesis manufacturers aim to improve their products all the time. (By the way, it's not a good idea to lose touch altogether with the hospital where you had your original operation, because they will hold your records. And in any case, it's advisable to keep going for checks from time to time.)

If you have had your operation in a private hospital, you will have to pay for your prosthesis, and the cost can be anything from £70 to £200. Some health insurance schemes make an allowance towards this expense, so it's worth making enquiries. Although there can be some regrettable lapses in the quality of the NHS service, it is still better than the no-service situation in many private hospitals. In the opinion of the experienced BCMA staff who hear many sad stories from their clients, women who opt for private treatment tend to receive even less advice and post-operative help than women who are treated under the NHS. However, even if you chose private health care for your first treatment, you can always opt to change to NHS treatment at a later stage.

## Choosing A Bra

I have already mentioned how important it is to wear the right size of bra. Too small is the usual problem, but it's equally important that your bra cup should not wrinkle or gape because it's too big. You may be lucky and find that you can still wear the same style that you had before your operation, but be prepared to make a change. This is where an experienced BCMA fitter can be a great help. She can advise you about the points you need to look out for in a bra, and tell you which among the big department stores offers the best range and service. Most of the large London stores and their branches have qualified mastectomy fitters and some, like Harrods, will provide an extra service by sewing pockets into bras and swimwear. Marks and Spencer, who are reputed to cup one in three bosoms in this country, will allow you to take bras home for trying on and return those which aren't right.

If you need pockets to be sewn into your bra you can have up to two a year done for you free of charge in some areas under the NHS. Others may make a small charge or no longer offer the service so it's important to ask what is available. Alternatively, if you are handy with your needle, you can sew wide tapes in the form of an 'X' across the back of the cup and slip the prosthesis behind them.

You may find it preferable to have a specially made mastectomy bra, which incorporates a pocket to hold your prosthesis. Again there is a good range available both through mail order and from specialist shops, some of which are listed in the Useful Addresses section. A complete list is available from the BCMA.

It's worth knowing that VAT is not payable on breast prostheses, mastectomy bras or mastectomy swimsuits. This exemption only applies to garments that have been specially made for women who have had breast surgery, so you can't apply for it when you buy ordinary clothing. Most shops supplying mastectomy wear will offer you a VAT exemption form to fill in, but if there's any possibility that they may not have them on the premises, take one of your own with you. You can copy this one out of the book or apply for forms from the BCMA. The form has to be completed at the time of buying the goods, otherwise you lose your right to the exemption. It's the shop's responsibility to forward the form to HM Customs and Excise in place of VAT.

---

### VAT EXEMPTION FROM

I (Full name)..............................................................................

Of (Address)..............................................................................

.................................................................................................

declare that I have had a Mastectomy and the goods mentioned below are being supplied to me for my personal use - Prosthesis/Bras/Swimwear (Delete as appropriate). I claim that the supply of these goods is eligible for relief from Value Added Tax under Group 14 of Schedule 4 to the Finance Act, 1972.

Signature...................................................................................

Date ..........................................................................................

---

# Beautiful And Brave

Everyone who was in the Great Ballroom at Grosvenor House Hotel on Thursday afternoon, 5th March 1992, probably felt the same – enchanted and deeply moved. They were watching thirteen elegant women, most of them middle-aged or older, gliding up and down the catwalk, showing off the new season's designer labels with the utmost poise and confidence as if they had been doing nothing else all their lives. The theme was holidays and they looked great in everything from sassy swimwear to floaty negligees; the fashion show culminated in a dazzling ballgown parade.

The occasion was a triumph. It was also unique because every one of those models had had surgery for breast cancer. And all the clothes they displayed with such style were off-the-peg. Nothing had been specially made for the occasion and everything fitted perfectly – no concealing capes or long sleeves or pleats and tucks here and there. No concessions, yet each woman looked better than good. She looked wonderful.

> 'I always wear off-the-peg lingerie but it took me years to go into a shop and explain without feeling embarrassed. I found it specially hard when I was looking for a bra, having to explain to the saleswoman. If this show helps one woman get over that quickly, it will be worthwhile.'
>
> *Helen*

That, of course, was the main reason for the BCMA fashion show – to help other women in the same position regain their confidence. It is just another expression of the organization's ethos that only women who have been through the experience of surgery for breast cancer can really help in practical ways other women coping with similar problems.

Showing it can be done – you can wear strapless dresses and plunging necklines if that's what you want, take vigorous exercise or sunbathe in a bikini – is infinitely more encouraging when it comes from another woman like yourself rather than from an advisor or friend, however well-meaning, who nonetheless hasn't 'been there' herself.

> 'At first I could not look at myself in the mirror and would wear only loose, cover-up clothes. Recently I've gained confidence, and this show is helping tremendously.'
>
> *Ouida*

The fashion show was the brainchild of Jinty Blanckenhagen, the former Director of the BCMA who, a few years earlier in America, had seen a so-called mastectomy fashion show where the models were standard issue – tall, slim and double-breasted – yet they were exhibiting 'mastectomy styles'. We can surely do better than this, thought Jinty, and immediately started working out how. It should be the other way round, she decided: women with mastectomies and other kinds of breast surgery should wear off-the-peg fashion, thus proving that life can and does return to normal. She gathered together a group of BCMA volunteers, including a former model and a dancer who were willing to follow her lead. These formed the nucleus and, with the help of friends in the fashion business, a year later the BCMA put on its first fashion show in Dublin, a success which was soon followed by others in Manchester, Glasgow and then this last glitzy one in London. More are planned for the future, as a kind of ongoing countrywide roadshow, with the hope that while individual women will be encouraged to feel better about themselves, other services provided by the BCMA will become better known as a result.

The beachwear collection is always a high spot of the show.

Women want to be able to swim and enjoy their holidays as before, but the thought of parading in a minimal bathing suit can be quite daunting. Don't let the fear of looking different or perhaps losing your prosthesis put you off. With a little ingenuity you will be able to secure your prosthesis and look exactly the same as you have always done. In fact, as long as your surgery has not been too extensive you may even be able to continue doing what you've always done.

> 'The first time I went on holiday after the operation I felt a bit nervous about going topless but I soon forgot about it. The suntan hid the scar.'
>
> *Katrina, who had a lumpectomy*

What you wear is obviously dictated by the kind of surgery you have had, but there are many clever things you can do with a bikini top to hide a scar and fill out the cup. You can drape it like a bandeau or choose one with a halter neck which gives you automatic uplift. You may prefer to wear a one-piece suit and sew a Cumfie or a trimmed synthetic sponge into the cup. If you use a sponge, always press your arm against the cup after swimming to remove as much water as possible. These are lightweight alternatives to your everyday prosthesis. Some manufacturers also make special prostheses for swimming, or you may prefer to buy a specially-made mastectomy swim suit from one of the specialist shops.

## Looking After Your Hand And Arm

As we have said in earlier chapters, it's important to look after the hand and arm on the same side as the operated breast. You will want to start exercising them as soon as possible after your operation so that you can recover your full mobility, but don't rush at it. In hospital the physiotherapist will take you through some exercises for strengthening your hand and arm muscles, and it's important that you follow her instructions carefully and continue these exercises when you get home. You may find them quite uncomfortable to begin with, so take it easy and do them little and often, gradually increasing the number of times a day until you feel your strength and mobility has returned.

The exercises illustrated here are taken from a free leaflet published by the BCMA. Before you start doing them, please check with your doctor that they are all suitable for you. Keep this book in a handy place so that you don't forget to do them. Alternatively, you could ask the BCMA to send you a leaflet which you can pin up on a notice board or on your dressing table mirror.

## HAND AND ARM EXERCISES

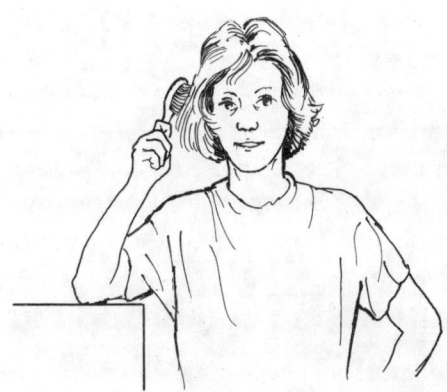

**Fig 14 Hair-brushing exercise** *(for hospital)*
*Rest elbow on bed-table. Keep head erect. Start by brushing one side only, then gradually increase to whole head. Don't overdo, but be persistent.*

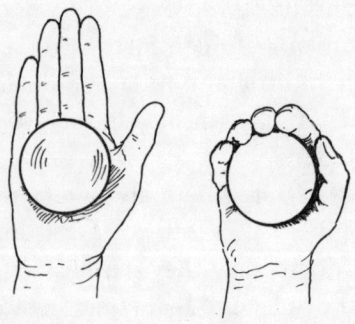

**Fig 15 Squeezing and relaxing hand** *(for hospital)*
*A rubber ball or similar object may be used.*

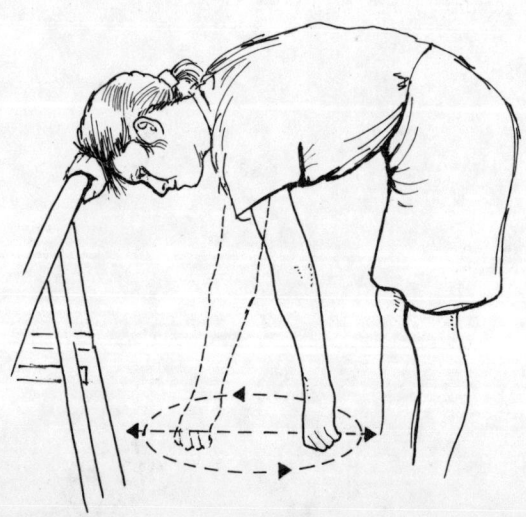

**Fig 16 Arm-swinging**
*Place unaffected arm on back of chair and rest forehead on arm. Allow your other arm to hang loosely and swing from shoulder, forwards and backwards, then side to side and in small circles. As arm relaxes, increase length of swings and size of circles. Swing until arm is relaxed.*

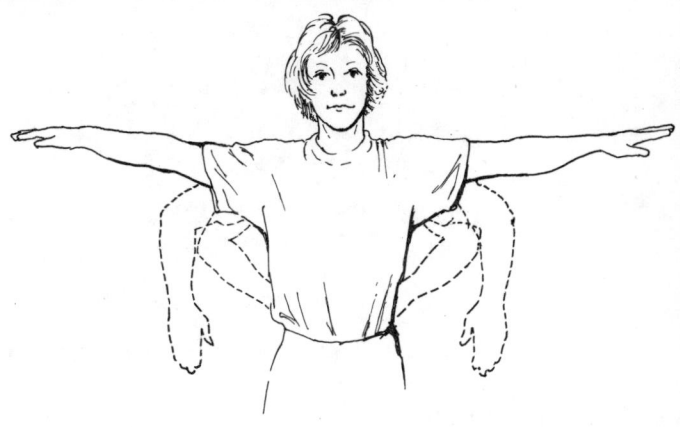

**Fig 17  Bra-fastening**
*Extend arms, drop hands from elbows, then slowly reach behind back to bra level.*

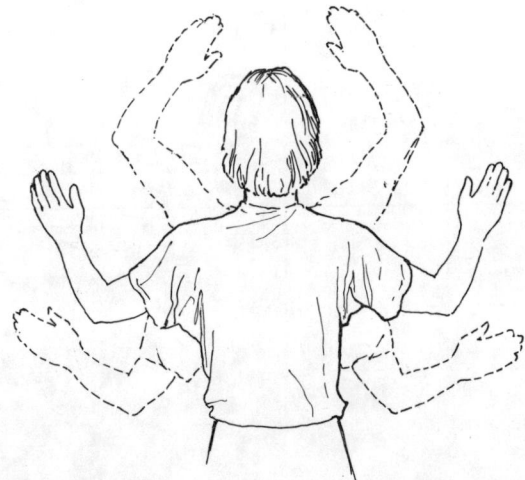

**Fig 18  Wall-reaching**
*Feet apart for balance. Stand close to and facing wall, Start with hands at shoulder level and gradually work hands up the wall. Slide hands back to shoulder level before starting exercise again. Do slowly several times a day. Mark spot reached and aim higher each time.*

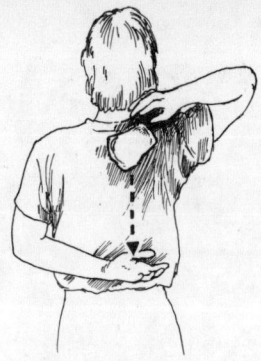

**Fig 19 Bean-bag exercise** *(a small purse or cosmetic bag will do just as well)*
*Drop bag from right hand over right shoulder into left hand at back. Repeat five times and do with opposite side.*

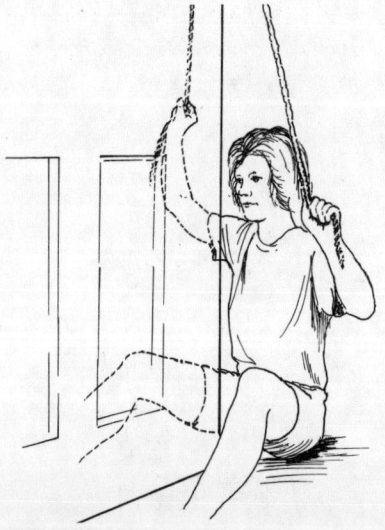

**Fig 20 Rope-pulley exercise**
*Throw rope or dressing gown cord over top of open door. Sit with door between legs. Hold lower end in hand on the side of your surgery and gently pull other end. Raise arm as high as possible each time, until full elevation.*

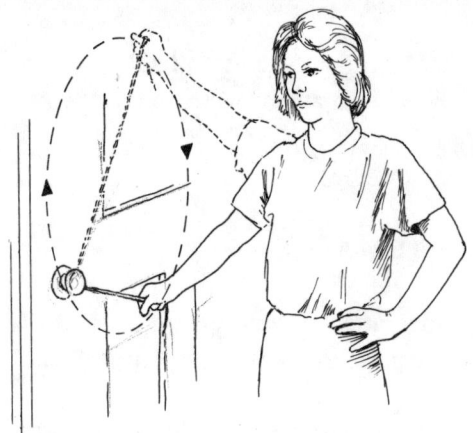

**Fig 21  Rope/string exercise**
*Attach rope to doorknob or handle. Make small circles with rope moving entire arm from the shoulder. Do five times in one direction and five times in the other and gradually increase size of circle (by moving in closer) and number of circles.*

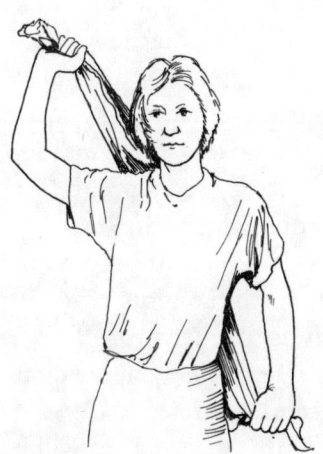

**Fig 22  Back-drying exercise**
*With towel or similar item use a gentle back-drying motion. Reverse procedure.*

# Problems

'Very few women get away with having no problems at all after surgery. They may not be serious but you do need help and support.'

*Helen*

## LYMPHOEDEMA

We have already referred to this problem in chapters five and seven. Lymphoedema, or 'heavy arm' as it's often called, is a condition which may develop some time after your operation or your course of radiotherapy. (See page 113 for the cause and precautions you can take to prevent lymphoedema occurring). Unfortunately, however careful you are, it's not always possible to prevent it. If you are unlucky and your arm does start to swell and redden and feel as if it's burning, it's important that you seek medical advice as soon as possible.

Regrettably, doctors in the UK tend to be rather apathetic about lymphoedema, taking the view that since the condition can't be reversed, the patient has just got to learn to live with it. French and German doctors take a much more positive attitude. While it is true that the condition is long-term and not curable, they have devised a programme of massage, skin care, exercise and diet which can keep it well under control. There are a few NHS clinics, most notably one at the Royal Free Hospital in north London, where this treatment is offered specifically to women who have had breast surgery. A small number of private lymphoedema clinics are also appearing (see Useful Addresses).

However, none of this external aid will be any good to you unless you play your part and take good care of yourself by following your physiotherapist's instructions carefully. It will mean wearing an elasticated support (compression) sleeve most of the time during the day and, at night, always sleeping with your arm laid on a pillow raised above your head to improve the drainage of excess fluid. It's vital to keep your skin moisturized and creamed, because the swelling makes it prone to cracking and dryness which can lead to infection. Even small cuts can harbour germs and the danger of repeated infections is that not only do they make you feel rotten, but they further weaken the lymphatic system in your arm. It's also important to do the exercises your therapist teaches you, because these are designed to help drain the fluid and prevent stiffness in your joints.

If you already have lymphoedema and are desperate to do something about it, you may find it a useful start to buy an excellent booklet called Lymphoedema by Claud Regnard, Caroline Badger and Peter Mortimer, available from the BCMA (price £2.50 including postage and packing). It's full of useful information and advice, and even if you can't get to a specialist clinic it may be worth showing it to your GP to help him or her understand your needs better and possibly enlist the help of a physiotherapist. Your GP can give you prescriptions for a compression sleeve, which will have to be replaced at regular intervals. A compression pump also works well for some women. It operates by gently squeezing and releasing the arm through an inflatable sleeve, but don't invest in the expense of getting one until you have discussed it with a lymphoedema therapist.

Whatever happens, don't despair about your condition. Although, at the beginning, improvement may seem intolerably slow, if you persist with your treatment programme, the swelling will slowly begin to ease and once you know what to do you will be able to keep the condition under control.

## SKIN BLEMISHES AND SCARS

Patches of discoloured skin can occur after radiotherapy and may not disappear altogether. The operation scars are sometimes higher than you would like. You can conceal them with cover creams, which come in shades to suit every skin colour. Details of manufacturers are on the BCMA stockist list. If you want advice about them, your local Red Cross office will be able to tell you which hospital in your area has a department dealing with these problems. You must ask your GP for a referral letter before you go to the hospital.

## LOCAL RECURRENCE

Sometimes the cancer reappears on the scar site, if you had a mastectomy, or close to the spot where the lump was removed in a lumpectomy. It usually looks like a small pink lump or lumps. Report it at once to your doctor who will be able to give you treatment for it. Usually a short course of radiotherapy is all that is necessary to bring it under control but sometimes, unfortunately, if you had a lumpectomy the first time, it may be necessary to have a mastectomy now.

It may not be cancer at all, but simply a necrosis of the scar tissue - literally a death of the tissue. This too can be treated quite easily, probably by a further small operation.

In general, always report any changes: in your other breast, under your arm or elsewhere in your body; or any symptoms like pain or a persistent cough. It may not be anything serious, but it's important that your doctor should be made aware of it as soon as possible. He or she is not going to think you are making an unnecessary fuss, and you could save yourself a lot of anxiety and further extended treatment by not letting things get out of control.

# 9

## *LIFE AFTER BREAST CANCER*

### A Strange Country

'When you are told you have breast cancer, you embark on a long journey in a strange and terrifying country whose farther boundaries are out of sight but whose inhabitants are helpful and kind . . . I believe that it is possible to live, and live well, with cancer.'

*Meredith, Daily Telegraph*, September 24, 1991

This chapter belongs to the women who have already been there, to this strange country with unmapped terrain through which each cancer patient has to find their own path. You could say that such a country is a metaphor for the life we all have to lead, with death, the invisible terminus, awaiting each one of us when we come round what is to be our final corner. The point about cancer is that it pulls you up short, often in the midst of life when you least expect it, and brutally reminds you of your mortality. There are no rules for a 'correct' response to that blow; your reactions can't be described as 'right' or 'wrong', they just are; and in the end, there will be no-one but you who can tell you how to proceed.

There is, all the same, great value in hearing about the experiences of others who have been down a similar path. They, better than anyone, can show you how it is possible to believe in yourself and your ability to overcome what may seem at first insuperable. They can also offer you genuine hope for the future, based on a realistic understanding of the present.

The women in this book have talked about how they felt when they first knew they had breast cancer; they have described how they coped with treatments and the changes it made in their physical wellbeing and their emotional state. Here they talk about the effect cancer has had on them in a more profoundly personal way: how it has changed their outlook and very often their aspirations; the influence it has had, often for the better, though not always, on their close relationships; the good things they have acquired from their experience as well as the sorrows and the pain it has brought them.

It takes time to assimilate an experience like cancer. Not every woman reading this book may find it possible within herself to be as positive and life-affirming as these women are, at least not immediately. But do remember, these women have all been down into the depths, and they have all emerged. They are the only people who can tell you what it feels like to live after breast cancer.

'Nothing quite prepared me for the shock of living. All those months of breast cancer treatment, crossing off the chemotherapy sessions in my diary, being cared for, suddenly came to an end. I stood outside the hospital, squinting into the December sunlight and wondered what to do next. It was pure joy mixed with blind panic. An affirmation of life combined with a sense of immense vulnerability.'

*Sheila, Observer*, October 13, 1991

Cancer changes your life. Before it happens you see your life from one perspective. Afterwards, you see it from another.

The new view may not necessarily be better than the old one, but the effect of cancer is to throw everything into sharp relief. And for many people life actually becomes more valuable and more enjoyable.

'One lingering side effect of treatment was an enhanced awareness of what makes life good. I feel as if I'm seeing places and people on a 22-inch state-of-the-art colour television instead of an old black-and-white portable.'

*Sheila, ibid.*

Your priorities change and so does your understanding of yourself. You appreciate as never before what you already have, all the good things in your life, and you realize that your future is not tomorrow but here and now, today.

'It wasn't a great shock to find I had cancer, but it did make me realize forcefully that this is not the dress rehearsal for life. This is it. I wake up each morning and celebrate the day ahead.'

*Jean*

Cancer can be a life-enhancing experience in many different ways. For one person it may make them thankful for what they have already got - a good job, a happy home life, recognition, material success or whatever else they count as important.

'It may seem a funny thing to say but my life is better for having had cancer. I've learnt so much from the experience - what my values are, who my friends are and how marvellous the good things of life are. You sift through the rubbish and quickly throw it out. After the diagnosis I kept saying to myself, I'm not ready yet, I've got so much to do still. Now, should I be run over by a bus tomorrow, I'll die happy because I've achieved everything I wanted. I've put my world right. I count my blessings every day.'

*Diana*

For another, cancer is the catalyst which makes them sit up and change the direction of their life. It could be their job, a relationship, or their own attitudes.

'Having cancer made me realize that I'd got into a rut. I did a course in music therapy and now I'm trying out various things to see what I really want to do. The cancer has given me a confidence which I never had before and it's made me aware that life is now. Hand in hand with the lows I have moments of feeling euphoric . . . so intensely alive it's wonderful.'

*Vera*

'I realized that he couldn't help me. My cancer frightened him too much. I didn't blame him but I ended the relationship because I knew he was only staying because he thought he should, and that was no good for me. I felt awful about it at the time but relieved as well. I didn't have the strength to cope with his problems as well as mine.

*Julia*

'I think much more about myself and what would upset me. I used to try hard to please others. Now I please myself and I avoid stress. I've realized that life is very short so I try to make the most of everything. You might never get the opportunity again.'

*Katrina*

Getting the most out of life, making it enjoyable and having fun is a high priority with many people who have had cancer.

'I don't sit and sorrow for myself. I still enjoy myself.'

*Una*

'The hardest time was when the treatment was finished but it was a very good time for re-evaluating and re-thinking my lifestyle. I did a degree which was terrific and after 14 years of paid employment it seemed like a rest cure. I made a conscious decision that I wasn't going to live to work, and that I wasn't going to knock myself out and get stressed and overtired. There were so many other things I wanted to do, like having long holidays with my daughter, singing, keeping fit, reading. Now I make time for them all. The main thing is to plan for nice things on a rolling basis, so you've always got something to look forward to and don't leave things undone.'

*Sue*

What some people call positive thinking and others a fighting spirit has always been intuitively regarded as likely to have a powerful effect on the outcome of cancer, especially by those who witness it in action: relatives and friends, for instance. We have probably all heard of, if not met, the person with life-threatening cancer who defies the medical prognosis and lives for years beyond what was expected or, in some rare cases, may even appear to be totally cured. This capacity to exert mind over matter has now been officially recognized by the medical profession, after doing some studies, of course. A few hospitals are now offering patients who show signs of clinical depression after cancer treatment a course in cognitive therapy which aims to help them shift into a more positive mental gear. Long-term results are not yet available, but it seems to be having a good effect.

Another name for this quality could be bloody-mindedness, and some people are naturally endowed with it. Such patients tend to be 'difficult' in the eyes of their doctors because they question everything, and aren't prepared to be compliant unless they are satisfied with the explanations being given to them. Bernie Siegel, an American surgeon who believes strongly that the body-mind connection promotes self-healing, calls them exceptional patients. Whatever the secret personality ingredient may be, it's quite definitely the reverse of being resigned or fatalistic. None of this 'your number's up' nonsense for these people.

'Faced by the shock of our mortality we all react differently. I experienced an icy determination to survive of such strength that I was literally high on will power. I left the hospital holding hands with my husband, who had been with me at every consultation.'

Meredith, *Daily Telegraph*, September 24, 1991

'I like to be told, even if it's bad. Then you can fight it. To me everything is a challenge.'

Ray

'Being told I had cancer didn't frighten me. I had a bloody good cry. I went straight from the hospital to pick up my daughter from the nursery and I was speechless, but then I became absolutely determined that it wasn't going to kill me . . . anyway, not yet.'

Sue

All the women quoted in this book believe that it is important to be open about cancer and that if you can talk about your situation frankly with as many people as possible, it's a great help. However, there are some people who cope extremely well by not talking about their cancer, perhaps not even acknowledging that they have had it. Who can tell exactly what they think about it, since they aren't willing to confide their feelings? Whatever you may think about the wisdom or otherwise of bottling up emotions, their point of view has to be respected, and their privacy should not be invaded. Each person with cancer has to find their own way of confronting their mortality and entering the battle for survival. One way of defending yourself is to put your feelings on ice, until you feel ready to handle them.

'I began to feel normal again when I started worrying. My feelings came out of hibernation when two friends were very ill earlier this year. All the fears and worries that I had refused to allow myself suddenly made sense for others.'
*Sheila, Observer*, October 13, 1991

One fear which almost all women find hard to admit to is their concern that the cancer may come back. It lurks at the back of their minds and each woman has to find her way of handling it.

'I don't think about it except when I'm ill and then I do worry it might've come back. I'd be a fool if I didn't.'
*Isobel*

'For a long time I thought about cancer every day. I don't do that any more, but I still have nightmares and the memory stays with me for days. You can't put it behind you completely but your way of coping with it does change. At the moment my energies are in counselling and working as a BCMA volunteer, because I know how much it meant to me to be able to talk to someone who knew what I was on about.'
*Vera*

The woman who has a loving and understanding partner is blessed. Many women find that after going through an initial upheaval, their relationship with their partner is deepened and strengthened. All the same, it's important not to take your family's support and strength for granted.

'As a mother you are so used to looking after the family, it can be very difficult for the family to look after you. They all need support, including the sisters and brothers of the patient. All the attention is focused on the woman; it's easy to forget that the partner goes through a very bad time too.'

*Ann*

Yet consideration for the needs of your family can impose strains on you.

'My sister and brother were very upset. I told them first, then I knew I had to tell my father. They came with me because they were very worried about how he'd take it. I saw him turn grey and he actually cried. But in his own way he has supported me. It's hard though and sometimes I still feel that I'm having to support them. I can't tell them everything.'

*Katrina, whose mother had died of breast cancer*

The mother of young or dependent children has her own private agonies to wrestle with. Will she live to see her children grow up? How can she explain to them what her illness means? Young children may be frightened or think that their mother's illness is a punishment because they've been naughty. Older children may feel burdened by the knowledge that it's cancer or angry with their mother because her illness is restricting them.

'The realization of just how much it matters for a mother to be there is very painful to me. I look at the children - extremely happy at the moment - and think: "Am I going to shatter their world by dying?"'

*Gillian, Guardian*, August 20, 1989

'At one time I didn't think I would see my children growing up. I'm now enjoying my grandson growing up.'

*Isobel*

Women in a relationship which is already fragile may find that cancer precipitates a crisis leading to breakdown. The crisis has simply exposed long-standing cracks, but a rupture at this point can have a devastating effect on a woman's emotional state. Many women fear sexual rejection because of their surgery, and anticipate their fear by rejecting their partner before he can do it to them. More often than not the fear is unfounded, but the partner finds it impossible to convince the woman. If you find yourself in a situation similar to this, either as partner or patient, don't be reluctant to seek help. There are organizations which are skilled at providing it (see chapter ten).

In most cases, though, the love of those who matter to you is warming and sustaining. You may even feel surprised by how much you mean to them. Cancer gives you an opportunity to tell them what they mean to you.

'It's no good looking over your shoulder. The only thing is to go forward. I no longer take my family for granted. I make darned certain they know how I feel about them and I never leave anything for tomorrow which I could do today.'

*Diana*

One thing you now know with absolute certainty is that nothing is ever going to be quite the same again. You can never go back to life as it used to be, nor may you wish to.

'I aim for optimum physical, mental and spiritual health. I never regret having cancer. It can be a good experience, teaching us to take stock of our lives. Everything is more beautiful to me now. I thank God daily for my life. I may not be alive this time next year but today, I know, I am happy.'

*Mary, Observer*, October 13, 1991

Life for all these women has genuinely taken on new meaning. Their experience has changed them, and they would say in most respects for the better, which in no way belittles the suffering they have had to endure. Like most other cancer patients, the one thing they don't want is pity or the impression that other 'normal' people see them as victims.

'The fact that I have had cancer is, I hope, one of the least interesting things about me. I refuse to be defined by the disease. I hate the image of the cancer survivor as plucky and forever smiling. I love life and look forward to my fortieth birthday next year. But I don't have to be Superwoman to prove I'm alive. I only have to open my eyes each morning.'

*Sheila, Observer*, October 13, 1991

# 10

## *ALWAYS A WOMAN*

It is rare for someone to be able to say with complete conviction that the experience of having cancer has made no difference to them. Cancer, as we have seen from the vivid testimonies in the last chapter, has a profound effect on most people. It would be surprising if it didn't, given its serious nature, but it shouldn't, as Sheila expressed with such fervour, define you as someone separate from the rest of the human race, nor should it be regarded as the most interesting thing about you. To think like that about anyone who has cancer is both patronizing and demeaning; to go further and convey that view to them reveals an appalling lack of imagination and can be deeply hurtful.

The women who have talked about their lives and their feelings in this book all believe that they have made more of themselves because they have had cancer. They and others like them may well feel that in some respects they have become better people for having had the experience, even if it's hard for them to describe precisely in what way this has happened. Those close to them may notice quite marked changes in attitudes and behaviour but none of these developments - interesting though they are, and some might call them signs of growth - turn them into people who are fundamentally different from how they were before their illness. The potential to be what they are today was always there within them. Cancer just happened to be the catalysing agent which has allowed that potential to flower.

Cancer is usually thought of as entirely destructive, 'the worm in the bud' which secretly eats away living tissue and takes with it the life harbouring it. As a bald description of cancer that is true enough, and as such, it has become, as Susan Sontag has written, a metaphor for all that is evil, and viciously underhand in our age. The medical need to cut the tumour out, and the mutilation resulting from that necessity, renders it even more of a spectre.

For the woman diagnosed with breast cancer, the threat of mutilation now confronting her seems particularly brutal because it is directed towards a part of her body which is a visible expression of her sexuality and her gender, an essential element in her total sense of being a woman. Although in most cases the fear of death outweighs the fear of mutilation, many women who are told they will need breast surgery become deeply distressed. Indeed, it would be rather strange if a woman faced with this prospect didn't feel some measure of unhappiness, whatever her age, since the loss or even semi-loss of a breast is a bereavement. As such it has to be mourned and the grief acknowledged, not just by her but by those caring for her. Her unhappiness is utterly comprehensible. Some discussion about how to cope with the emotions it generates has already been raised earlier in this book.

By the time you have reached this chapter, I hope you will be feeling that though the cancer you have is frightening and is serious - no one should minimize its gravity - you do have some weapons with which to fight it. For a start you have knowledge, a good deal more perhaps than when you began reading at page one. And you have been encouraged, I hope, by reading about other women's experiences and gained confidence thereby as well.

These women have done much more than survive. They

have come through their ordeal and they are living triumphantly - as complete women. They have been through the agony of facing up to breast surgery and the ensuing treatment, and each has made her personal pact with herself about how she handles that. Now that situation is behind them and they are moving forward through their life in the same way as everyone else does, along unmarked tracks through uncharted country, but maybe they are a little more positive and certainly a good deal braver than many of us.

'I hated the idea of losing my breast but I was even more terrified of death. I'm so grateful to be alive and I can honestly say I don't feel any less of a woman because I've only got one breast.'

*Joyce*

It makes a tremendous difference, obviously, if you are lucky enough to have a loving and supportive partner. The husband or lover who can physically show the woman he loves that a change in her body image hasn't changed his feelings for her, will be giving her the best possible tonic. (This is true, obviously, for lesbian relationships as well.) Even so, the loving partner may have to be prepared for it to take a while before the message sinks in and is really accepted.

'I think she thought I was saying her mastectomy made no difference to me just to please her. She used to come upstairs to bed after me when I was already asleep, or she'd spend ages in the bathroom. I could feel her stiffening if I came near her. It got so bad and it was upsetting both of us, so in the end we went to a marriage guidance counsellor and she helped us through it.'

*Peter*

This doesn't mean that all women without partners feel that they are lacking vital support in this intimate area of their lives. They may be getting plenty of loving hugs and comforting affection from their family and friends, or, they may prefer, quite genuinely, to deal quietly on their own with this problem. Perhaps they don't really see it as a significant problem: maybe they did suffer a painful sense of loss at the beginning, but they have their own way of dealing with it and they believe it's something they can get over. People with a strong religious belief may derive great strength from it at times like this. Others with similar beliefs may have an opposite reaction, feeling deceived and angry, in a sense personally affronted, as if God had deliberately let them down.

These are very private places in people's lives, and no one would want to intrude on them unless invited in, but sometimes the cries for help are faint and may go unheard. If you are feeling confused and unhappy and don't know who to turn to, it's important to know there are people and organizations who are there to offer you help and advice.

## Woman To Woman

When Betty Westgate had her mastectomy at the age of 49 in 1968, it was in the days when the subject of cancer was completely taboo. The doctor had told her the lump was benign so she was surprised a week later to receive an admittance-to-hospital form. She queried it, only to be told by an anonymous voice over the telephone: 'You've got breast cancer. We're taking it off next week.' She packed her bags but said not a word to her family about cancer. She wanted to spare her husband for as long as possible, because she knew how upset he would be; as for her mother, Betty said 'she'd have had me dead and buried before I'd even got into the operating theatre, so terrified was she of cancer'.

Betty made a good recovery and told her husband and sons what she had when they came to visit her in hospital. When it was all over and she had finished her course of radiotherapy, she went back to her job as a teacher. She recalls now with wry amusement her determination at the time that cancer wasn't going to change her life. However, she was prepared to talk about her experience, and that was quite unusual in those days. Her openness attracted other women in the same position to her. She thinks her work as a Samaritan probably helped.

'Because I'd had cancer, people felt they could talk more freely to me. I found they needed information and non-medical help. Using volunteers to help other women in the same situation just seemed common sense.' From Betty's simple observation that there was a need and that she had found a way of meeting it, by enlisting the help of other women who had been through a similar experience, sprung the organization that she called The Mastectomy Association and today is known as the Breast Care and Mastectomy Association.

She had intended it to remain locally based in the area of South London where she lived, but the letters started pouring in, following an article in the *Daily Telegraph* about her work. Soon it became a national organization, although Betty continued to finance and run it for several years single-handed with only the support of her devoted husband. Then the money started to come in, slowly at first, from a few wellwishers, families who were grateful for the help the Association had given them, and one doctor who believed in what she was doing. She made it a principle never to accept money from commercial organizations, nor would she charge for the talks which she was invited to give all over the country.

In 1977, after years of being cold-shouldered by the medical profession, recognition and more money began to come her way. The Department of Health gave her a small grant which was followed up in 1979 with funding from Cancer Relief to appoint an administrator. In 1978 she was awarded the MBE. In the early 1980s a full-time director was appointed and Betty took a back seat as President. Today, BCMA is almost wholly funded by Cancer Relief, and in 1991 was operating with an income of close to half a million pounds. It has three offices, one in London, one in Glasgow and one in Edinburgh; a Director in London who has a full-time staff of 12; and a countrywide volunteer network of more than 500 women.

BCMA offers two unique services, both started by Betty: first, there is the prosthesis advisory and fitting service which was described in chapter eight; and second, there is the volunteer network. Volunteers are organized into regional networks, supported, where possible, by a regional organizer. They are encouraged to meet regularly, to share information and to support each other. The other function of the networks is to raise the profile of the BCMA in the regions. By working together volunteers can publicize the service and make links with health professionals. There is a volunteer section based at the London office which coordinates the network and sets up training courses.

The BCMA is developing a wide range of voluntary activities with one-to-one emotional support being only one option for those becoming involved with the organization. Volunteers who give emotional support are selected and trained and must have had surgery at least two years earlier. This is to make sure that you have worked through your own difficulties as far as possible before you start attempting to help other women. Almost all the volunteers will have had surgery for breast cancer. Some will have had lumpectomies or other treatments, and just a few will be women whose surgery was for a benign condition. They are an assorted bunch, coming from all age groups and backgrounds: they may be housewives, grannies, career women, full-time Mums or in part-time employment. All of them have volunteered because they know what it's like to be on your own, with no one to talk to who can really understand what you are going through.

> 'I try to give encouragement through example, in as much as I can say "here I am, fit and well, after so many years."'
>
> *Sue*

> 'This nice woman didn't seem to mind what I told her. Almost the best thing she did for me was to tell me where I could find a decent bra.'
>
> *Lucy*

A volunteer is prepared to give any kind of practical information or emotional support a woman might need, and she will do this over the telephone or in hospital. Sometimes she will visit a woman at home if she particularly requests it, but the purpose of the network is not to strike up friendships. The volunteer gives her help as and when it's needed and then moves on. The one thing she must not do is make any attempt to give medical advice or information. However, if the client seems very distressed she may suggest that she seek psychiatric advice through her GP or, if it's clear that she has not understood her diagnosis or needs medical information of some kind, she will be strongly advised to return to her consultant.

In addition to these two special services, both offered completely free of charge, the BCMA has a Helpline open in office hours and staffed by experienced information officers. It also supplies, again free of charge, a full range of informative literature on all aspects of breast care and treatment for breast cancer and other breast conditions.

# Other Sources Of Help

Cancer Relief Macmillan Fund is a national charity working to improve the quality of life for people with cancer. Every year in one way or another it helps 150,000 people with cancer. Amongst its activities it funds the training of Macmillan nurses who work with cancer patients at home and in hospital, a number of whom are trained specifically as breast cancer nurses. It also funds a range of medical and academic posts to improve the health professionals' understanding of cancer. It builds in-patient and day care units for cancer patients to provide specialist care in comfortable, non-clinical settings. It also provides practical and financial help to cancer patients. On the information side, it funds four charities which provide information and self-help support to cancer patients.

CancerLink, which was started in 1984, is one of them, along with the BCMA, the British Colostomy Association and the National Association of Laryngectomee Clubs. In addition to its cancer Helpline and information literature, CancerLink acts as a coordinating centre for self-help support groups throughout the country, many of which have been started by breast cancer patients. If you wanted to join such a group in your area, or start one, it would be able to help you. CancerLink also runs training courses for group leaders.

BACUP, founded in 1985 and based in London, but with a Freeline which extends throughout the UK, was also started by a cancer patient, the redoubtable Dr Vicky Clement-Jones. Her intention (fully realized before she died) was to make it an information and support service available not just to patients with cancer but to their families and friends as well. These people, Vicky realized from her own experience, frequently get left out and forgotten because of the attention focused on the patient, yet are often in desperate need of help, support and information. BACUP runs a free telephone service staffed by ten cancer nurses which responds to 30,000 callers a year. It also offers one-to-one counselling by trained volunteer counsellors at their London base. It has an extensive range of excellent booklets on various types of cancer and treatments, and issues a free newspaper for cancer patients and their families – *BACUP News* – three times a year (all free).

Aspect is the new informal name of the charity registered as The Jeannie Campbell Breast Cancer Radiotherapy Appeal. This organization publishes free booklets and factsheets about various aspects of breast cancer, especially those concerning modern conservational techniques.

These and other organizations which either provide information and support for cancer patients or promote cancer research are fully listed in the Useful Addresses section.

Breast cancer is a frightening disease, but I hope that by the time you have reached the final page of this book you will at least no longer be feeling alone and unsupported. If this book has helped you in any way at all, please lend it or pass it on to someone else who may need it.

# Useful Addresses

This is a selection of the main manufacturers of prostheses, bras and swimwear who will send you brochures and other information on request. For a complete and up-to-date list of retail stockists throughout the country write to the BCMA at its London office enclosing an sae. (For address see **useful organizations** below.)

**Abella International Ltd. (Anita)**, Anita Advisory Service, 3rd Floor, Scottish Provident House, 76-80 College Road, Harrow, Middlesex HA1 1DF
Tel. 081-427 9611

**Amoena (UK) Ltd.**, 18 Monks Brook Park, School Close, Chandlers Ford, Eastleigh, Hampshire SO5 3RA
Tel 0703 270345

**Rita Eaton**, 12 Brancaster Close, Leicester, LE4 0LA
Tel. 0533 352247

**Nicola Jane**, Mare Hill, Pulborough, West Sussex, RH20 2DY
Tel. 07982 2298/2784

**Medimac Ltd.**, 57 Kings Barn Lane, Steyning, West Sussex, BN4 3YR
Tel. 0903 816242

**Spencer Limited (Silima)**, Spencer House, Britannia Road, Banbury, Oxon, OX16 8DP
Tel. 0295 257301

**Trulife Limited**, 9/15 Grundy Street, Liverpool L5 9YH
Tel. 051-207 5690

# Useful Organizations

Listed below, and grouped by country, are national organizations offering information, support and practical help. There may be local groups in your area whose details you can get from one of the national information services or from your family doctor or the hospital.

## ENGLAND, SCOTLAND AND WALES

**Aspect (The Jeannie Campbell Breast Cancer Radiotherapy Appeal)**, 29 St Luke's Avenue, Ramsgate, Kent CT11 7JZ
Tel. 0843 596732
Promotes knowledge of breast-saving techniques and distributes free leaflets on various treatments.

**The Association of Sexual and Marital Therapists**, PO Box 62, Sheffield S10 3TS
Will send list of centres offering treatment for sexual problems and also list of individual therapists.

**BACUP (The British Association of Cancer United Patients)**, 3 Bath Place, London EC2A 3JR
Tel. Cancer Information Service 071-613 2121
Freeline (outside 071 and 081 areas) 0800 181199 (10-7 Mon-Thurs. 10-5.30 Fri).
Cancer Counselling Service 071-696 9000
Administration 071-696 9003

Telephone helplines are run by cancer nurses and are open to anyone seeking information or help about anything to do with any cancer. BACUP has more than 40 booklets describing treatments for most of the main types of cancer and other aspects of coping. Three times a year it publishes a free newspaper (BACUP News) to which patients, relatives or friends are welcome to contribute.

**BCMA (Breast Care & Mastectomy Association)**, 15/19 Britten Street, London SW3 3TZ
  Tel. Help and information line 071-867 1103
  Administration 071-867 8275
  Suite 2/8, 65 Bath Street, Glasgow G2 2BX
  Tel. 041-353 1050
  511 Lanark Road, Edinburgh, EH14 5DQ
  Tel. 031-458 5598 (9-12.30 Answering machine other times)
A woman-to-woman network with more than 500 volunteers helping women to cope before, during and after their treatment for breast cancer. Information staff give non-medical information, emotional support and practical advice over telephone. Free fitting service for prostheses, bras and swimwear in all the offices, by appointment only. Will send up-to-date list of stockists on request and also has a good range of free illustrated publications written specially for women diagnosed with breast cancer.

**Bristol Cancer Help Centre**, Grove House, Cornwallis Grove, Clifton, Bristol BS8 4PG
  Tel. 0272 743216
Runs residential and daytime courses in various complementary therapies for cancer sufferers.

**British Lymphoedema Clinics**, Part of BM Ltd., Suite 506, Britannia House, 9 Glenthorne Road, London W6 0LF
  Tel. 081-748 3791

Private clinics in London and Oxford offering manual lymph drainage, compression bandaging and hosiery, plus free advice and support.

**BUPA**, Women's Screening Unit, Battle Bridge House, 300 Gray's Inn Road, London WC1X 8DU
Tel. 071-278 4651 or 071-837 6484
Appointments 071-837 7055
Offers a complete well woman check-up. Also has mobile breast screening units in various regions. Fees and further information on request.

**CancerLink**, 17 Britannia Street, London WC1X 9JN
Tel. Information service 071-833 2451
For Groups Support Service and all other calls
Tel. 071-833 2818
9 Castle Terrace, Edinburgh, EH1 2DP
Tel. 031-228 5557 (Weekdays 10-5. Answering machine other times)
Provides information and support on all aspects of cancer. Acts as a resource centre to cancer support and self-help groups and helps people wishing to start a new group. Free publications.

**CARE (Cancer Aftercare and Rehabilitation Society)**, 21 Zetland Road, Redland, Bristol BS6 7AH
Tel. 0272 427419
An organization of cancer patients, relatives and friends who offer help and support. Branches throughout the country.

**Cancer First Aid**, 49 Westbourne Gardens, London W2 5NR
Tel. 071-221 0227/1796
Provides financial aid to cancer patients and their dependants who are suffering financial problems as a result

of illness. Grant applications are processed within 48 hours and paid direct to the claimant.

**Cancer Relief Macmillan Fund**, 15/19 Britten Street, London SW3 3TZ
  Tel. 071-351 7811
Funds training of Macmillan nurses to care for cancer patients both in hospital and at home. Also gives grants to people in financial difficulties because of their illness and funds a range of medical posts to improve health professionals' knowledge and practice of cancer care.

**ICM (The Institute for Complementary Medicine)**, 4 Tavern Quay, Sweden Gate, Surrey Quays, London SE16 1QZ
  Tel. 071 237 5165
Library, information about professional associations in complementary medicine, funds research and publishes the *Journal of Complementary Medicine.*

**Marie Curie Cancer Care**, 28 Belgrave Square, London SW1X 8QG
  Tel. 071-235 3325
Provides medical care for cancer patients through 5,000 community nurses and in 11 hospices.

**Tenovus Cancer Information Centre**, 142 Whitchurch Road, Cardiff CF4 3JN
  Tel. Information 0222 619846
  Bilingual helpline 0222 691998
Provides cancer information and support services for patients, their families and self-help groups. Also raises £2 mllllon a year to fund research into various cancers including breast.

**Women's Health**, 52-54 Featherstone Street, London EC1Y 8RT
  Tel. 071-251 6580

Provldes advice and information and puts women in touch with health care organizations throughout the country. Library and newsletter.

**Women's Health Concern**, 83 Earls Court Road, London W8 6ER
Tel. 071-938 3932
Advises women on all aspects of health with particular emphasis on menopause and related problems. Counselling and publications.

**Women's Nationwide Cancer Control Campaign**, Suna House, 128 Curtain Road, London EC2A 3AR
Tel. Helpline 071-729 2229
Pioneered mobile breast screening units. Educates women in value of screening for breast and cervical cancer but will answer other queries as well.

**NORTHERN IRELAND**
**Ulster Cancer Foundation**, 40-42 Eglantine Avenue, Belfast BT9 6DX
Tel. 0232 663281
Funds a mastectomy advisory service coordinator who runs a mastectomy centre at head office similar to the BCMA service. She also liaises between volunteers and support groups.

**AUSTRALIA**
Miss Anne Fletcher, Queensland Cancer Fund, William Rudder House, PO Box 201, Springhill, Queensland.
Tel. 612 257 1155

**CANADA**
William K. Adair, Director Service to Patients, Canadian Cancer Centre, 77 Bloor Street, Suite 1702, Toronto, Ontario, M5S 3A1

**NEW ZEALAND**
Miss Betty Krebs, National Coordinator Breast Cancer
Support Service, 121 Moxham Avenue, Wellington 3
  Tel. 644 863 349

**SOUTH AFRICA**
Mr J. P. F. Delport, National Cancer Association of South
Africa, 9 Jubilee Road, Parktown, PO Box 2000,
Johannesburg
  Tel. 447484

**Reach to Recovery** was founded in 1970 to help women
with breast cancer. Today it acts as an advisory and
coordinating body to the many breast cancer organizations
from all over the world which are affiliated to it. For further
information contact: Mrs Francine Timothy, International
Coordinator, 3 Rue Philibert Delorme, 75017 Paris, France.
  Tel. 46 22 02 83

# Further Reading

**BREAST CANCER**
Baum, Michael and Saunders, Christobel, *Breast Cancer - The Facts*, Oxford University Press (3rd edition) 1993.
Cirket, Cath, *Breast Awareness*, Thorsons, 1992.
Cochrane, John and Szarewski, Dr Anne, *The Breast Book*, Macdonald Optima, 1989.
Fallowfield, Lesley, and Clark, Andrew, *Breast Cancer*, Tavistock/ Routledge, 1991.
Gilbert, Dr Patricia, *What Every Woman Should Know About Her Breasts*, Sheldon Press, 1986.
Lorde, Audrey, *The Cancer Journals*.
Moran, Diana, *A More Difficult Exercise*, Bloomsbury, 1989.

**CANCER IN GENERAL**
Clyne, Rachel, *Cancer - Your Life, Your Choice*, Thorsons, 1989.
Kfir, Nira, and Slevin, Maurice, *Challenging Cancer - from chaos to control*, Routledge, 1991.
LeShan, Lawrence, *Cancer as a Turning Point*, Gateway Books, 1990.
Shaw, Clare, and Hunter, Maureen, *The Cancer Special Diet Cookbook*, Thorsons 1991.
Siegel, Bernie S., *Love, Medicine and Miracles*, Rider, 1988 and *Peace, Love and Healing*, Harper & Row, 1989.

Sikora, Professor Karol, and Thomas, Dr Hilary, *Fight Cancer*, BBC Books, 1989.

Williams, Chris and Sue, *Cancer: a Guide for Patients and Their Families*, Wiley, 1986.


## COMPLEMENTARY MEDICINE

Bishop, Beata, *A Time to Heal*, Severn House, 1985.

Brohn, Penny, *Gentle Giants*, Century, 1986.

Courtenay, Anthea, *Healing Now*, J. M. Dent & Sons, 1991.

Fulder, Stephen, *How to be a healthy patient - a holistic guide to medical treatment*, Headway, 1991.

Olsen, Kristin, *The Encyclopedia of Alternative Health Care*, Piatkus, 1989.

Wylie, Philip, *The Holistic Network Directory*.


**References** for the major medical papers referred to in the text are as follows:

'Systemic treatment of early breast cancer by hormonal, cytotoxic, or immune therapy, Parts I and II', Early Breast Cancer trialists' Collaborative Group, *The Lancet*, 4 and 11 January 1992, 339.

'Attitudes to chemotherapy: comparing views of patients with cancer with those of doctors, nurses, and general public', Maurice L. Slevin, et al. *BMJ* 2 June 1900, 300, 1458-1460.

'Effect of Psychosocial Treatment on Survival of Patients with Metastatic Breast Cancer', David Spiegel, Joan R. Bloom, Helena C. Kraemer, Ellen Gottheil, *The Lancet*, October 14, 1989 plus correspondence in issues dated 18th November and 16th December (reply from Spiegel).

# Glossary

**Adjuvant** auxiliary or additional. Term applied to any therapy which is used as back-up to primary treatment (usually surgery) of primary tumour. Chemotherapy, radiotherapy and hormone therapy can all be used as adjuvants.

**Aetiology** scientific enquiry into the causes of disease.

**Axilla** armpit; hence **axillary**, relating to the armpit.

**Benign breast disease** an umbrella term for a variety of non-malignant breast disorders, although some may be painful and require treatment.

**Biopsy** the surgical removal of a small piece of tissue for laboratory examination by a pathologist to determine whether it is malignant. **Excision biopsy** the surgical removal of a whole breast lump, usually done under general anaesthetic. The results of laboratory testing and analysis will take a few days.

**Carcinogen** any agent which causes cancer.

**Chemotherapy** the use of one or more anti-cancer (cytotoxic) drugs to destroy cancer cells. Can be used as first-line treatment to shrink tumour or, more usually, as adjuvant therapy to destroy any cancer cells which may have spread from the primary site into other parts of the body. Also used to control recurrence. **Combination chemotherapy** describes the use of several anti-cancer drugs in varying proportions to treat early and advanced cancer. This is based on the principle that their combined use will improve their effectiveness and reduce toxicity.

**Complementary medicine** wide variety of therapies ranging from acupuncture to Zen meditation which fall outside orthodox medical range but can be used to supplement cancer treatments. Sometimes called 'alternative' or 'natural'.

**Clinical medicine** medical practice based on observed symptoms; hence **clinical examination** for breast disease is the physical examination of a patient's breast, and **clinical staging** is diagnosing the extent of cancer by analysing the conclusions drawn from the examination.

**Cyst** an accumulation of material, usually fluid, contained in a sac. It is a common non-malignant condition, especially in women approaching the menopause, and is only rarely associated with a cancer.

**Cytology** microscopic examination of individual or groups of cells.

**Cytotoxic** means substance poisonous to cells. Term applied to drugs used in chemotherapy to describe their anti-cancer effect.

**Diagnosis** formal identification of a disease by its symptoms.

**Ductal carcinoma in situ (DCIS)** a small contained tumour in one of the breast ducts which, if removed at this early stage before it has spread, virtually assures cure.

**Endocrine or hormone therapy** treatment controlling hormone activity in tumours suspected to be hormone-dependent.

**Endogenous** growing or originating from within the body.

**Epidemiology** science of epidemics and now of disease generally.

**Exogenous** growing or originating from outside the body.

**Fine-needle aspiration** a technique to differentiate cystic from solid lesions in the breast. A needle is inserted in the lesion and the material drawn out with a syringe. If the material is solid it can be stained and the cells are examined in a laboratory to determine whether or not they are malignant. This technique is known as **Fine-needle aspiration cytology**.

**Frozen section** small piece of suspect tissue which is cut out (excised) at biopsy, frozen, and sent for immediate pathological examination.

**Gamma rays** a type of electromagnetic radiation with wavelengths shorter than those of X-rays. They therefore carry more energy than X-rays and when used for radiotherapy deliver more energy to tumours, except for those X-rays now delivered by a linear accelerator, which has energies of several million volts.

**Histology** science of organic tissues; hence **histologic analysis** is examining tissue for changes caused by disease, and **histologic classification** is naming and determining the extent and type of disease.

**Holistic medicine** considers the whole person, physically, psychologically and culturally, rather than treating merely the diseased part. Can be practised both by orthodox medical practitioners and complementary therapists.

**Hormone** a chemical substance, produced in certain parts of the body, which has a specific effect on the activity of one or more distant organs.

**Hormone Replacement Therapy (HRT)** treatment of menopausal and post-menopausal women who are given natural oestrogen by tablet, injection, patch or implant to replace the oestrogen deficiency which is the natural result of the ovaries ceasing to function.

**Hysterectomy** removal of the uterus; depending on the reason for surgery, other reproductive organs like cervix, fallopian tubes and ovaries may also be removed.

**Immunology** scientific study of resistance to infection in humans and animals. Hence **immunological** responses describe ways in which the body defends itself against disease; **immunosuppressive** refers to any agent which prevents these defence mechanisms from operating; and **immunotherapy** is treatment based on principle of supporting or improving the body's natural defence mechanisms.

**Implant** artificial substance, usually silicone gel, which is inserted into breast cavity to replace the natural breast.

**Invasive cells** are cells that grow inwards, changing normal body tissue into abnormal, cancerous tissue.

**Interval cancer** a cancer that is diagnosed because of symptoms within a stated interval after a negative screening test.

**Ionizing radiation** energy emitted as electromagnetic waves, used in radiotherapy and X-ray diagnosis. Must be used with care, as heavy or too many repeated applications can cause cancer.

**Lesion** changes in the functioning or texture of an organ which is caused by disease.

**Local recurrence** cancer which reappears on site of original tumour. Hence **local therapy** is treatment applied directly to this site.

**Lumpectomy** the most conservative form of mastectomy, involving removal of malignant tumour only in the breast, together with small amount of surrounding tissue.

**Lymph** colourless fluid from body tissue and organs which resembles blood but has no red corpuscles.

**Lymph gland or node** small mass of tissue found in clusters all over the body in which lymph is purified and **lymphocytes** (colourless blood cells) are formed. In breast cancer, the condition of the **axillary, pectoral** and **mammary** nodes which surround the breast is an important indication for prognosis about the extent of cancer spread.

**Lymphoedema** swelling of the arm caused by fluid which cannot drain away normally because the lymphatic drainage system - i.e. the lymph nodes - have been removed, either surgically or by irradiation.

**Malignant** in cancer refers to growths which will spread, ultimately with fatal results, if not removed.

**Mamma** or mammary gland milk-secreting organ of female mammals; in women called the breast.

**Mammography** X-ray diagnostic technique specially developed to investigate the breast for cancer cells.

**Mastectomy** surgical procedure to remove the breast. (For description of various types see text).

**Menarche** first menstruation

**Menopause** (often called 'the change'). Period of life, usually between forty-five and fifty-five, when a woman ceases to menstruate, signifying the end of her reproductive life.

**Metastasis** the process by which malignant cells detach themselves from the primary tumour and establish themselves in distant parts of the body, starting new tumours called **metastases** or **secondaries**. If they are so small that they can't be detected they are called **micro-metastases**.

**Morbidity** diseased state of organ or tissue.

**Neoplasia** cancer; hence **neoplasm** malignant tumour and **neoplastic** of, or relating to, malignant tumours.

**Node-positive** describes condition of one or more lymph nodes which have been diagnosed as invaded by cancer cells.

**Nulliparous** describes woman who has never given birth to a child.

**Occult carcinoma** a small tumour which is asymptomatic (gives no indicatlon of its presence).

**Oncology** the study of the causes, development, characteristics and treatment of cancer; hence **oncologist**

doctor who specializes in cancer treatment (usually a surgeon, physician or radiotherapist).

**Oopherectomy** procedure, either by surgery or radiation, to remove the ovaries, sometimes called **ovarian ablation** or **castration**.

**Pathologist** specialist in laboratory medicine concerned to identify the changes in body tissues and organs which cause or are caused by disease.

**Pituitary gland**, also known as the **hypophysis**. A small organ at the base of the brain which is responsible for synthesizing and releasing at least nine different hormones. Exerts important influence on growth and bodily functions.

**Prognosis** medical prediction about the development of a disease diagnosed in a patient.

**Prolactin** hormone, secreted by the pituitary gland, which stimulates the milk flow.

**Prophylactic** medical action to prevent disease.

**Prosthesis** artificial part to replace some portion of the human anatomy. Where there has been a mastectomy, the term applies equally to surgical implants and to manufactured breast forms, usually made of silicone, which are worn inside the bra cup.

**Punch biopsy** very small piece of tissue cut out to be tested.

**Radiographer** professionally trained person who takes radiographs and is involved with other imaging techniques.

**Radiologist** specialist concerned with the diagnosis of disease by means of imaging techniques.

**Radiotherapy** treatment of cancer by ionizing radiation, which is energy emitted as electromagnetic waves to destroy the malignant cells; hence **radiotherapist** doctor who plans radiotherapy treatment.

**Radium** radioactive metallic element derived from pitchblende, sometimes used in radiotherapy.

**Remission** a period of good health occurring after the onset of cancer or following recurrence. It can happen spontaneously or be induced by treatment.

**Scan** detailed picture of structures inside the body taken either with X-rays (computerized tomography – CT) or using magnetism (magnetic resonance imaging – MRI) or with high-frequency sound waves (ultrasound).

**Secondaries** recurrence of cancer cells in distant parts of the body after discovery of the primary tumour.

**Tumour** swelling mass of tissue in any part of the body, derived from pre-existing cells, which serves no purpose and grows independently of surrounding tissue. **Benign tumours** remain localized, are usually slow-growing and produce symptoms only when their size interferes with surrounding tissue. **Malignant tumours** have varying rates of growth but eventually, if left untreated, they tend to invade surrounding tissue and spread to other parts of the body.

**Ultrasonography** production of a visual image of deep structures of the body by recording the echoes of sound waves directed into the tissues.

# Index